Tai Chi Chuan

The Fundamentals

基本面太极拳

Author – Sifu Bob

Table of Contents

Preface

This is the first of a series of Tai Chi Chuan volumes from Golden Flower Internal Arts. This is a volume focusing on the basic understanding of the fundamentals of Tai Ch'i Chuan. This volume is also focused on the Yang form that followed from the connection with Yang Chen Fu. The volume has limited illustrations for a reason. The basic ideas of Tai Ch'i Chuan the same but are when looking at each school play a form their interpretation will be different. The idea of this volume is to make the fundamentals readable and not arguable. Use this volume for the information it can pass on.

After this volume, the next volume is focused on the deeper theory of Tai Ch'i Chuan with the focus on the the original principles handed down from the early masters. The volume is extensive and also not relying on pictures but to discuss the theory of the art.

The next three volumes are focused on the Cheng Man Ching School as handed down through Grandmasters Chen and Liang. There is a form volume that breaks down all the movements in a form with the aid of pictures. This will provide guidance of applying the principles of the basics and the theory of Tai Ch'i Chuan. Two other volumes are focused on the application of Tai Ch'i Chuan – not necessary for a fighting purpose but as a martial art. One will be on Tui Shou and the other on San Shou.

Note: This volume is being published at the beginning of the Pandemic. The volume is rushed to be sure that it is published and we apologize for the lack of pictures. We believe that the content is worth publishing at this time. The other volumes provide adequate pictures and diagrams.

Dedication

To all my many teachers

Grandmaster William C. C. Chen

Grandmaster Liang Tse Tung

Master Chan Bun-Piac

Dr. John P. Painter

Thomas Morgan – asking the questions and challenging the answers.

And the many more

Remember as T.T. always said "you need teachers and you need books" and now maybe videos … coming soon?

Copyright

Text and Pictures

Copyright © 2016 Robert G. Downey

All Rights Reserved

Public domain Photos from Gray's Anatomy

(If you don't have a volume get one!)

The information in this book is provided as a service to the general public. While the information in this book is about exercise, health, and lifestyle issues, it is not intended as medical or health advice or as a substitute for medical care or consultation. Understand that your practice of any exercises or examples, dietary practices or food, drink or nutritional supplements carries with it the potential for certain risks, some of which may not be reasonably foreseeable and requires your consideration of the impact on your health. Always seek the advice of your doctor with any questions you may have regarding a medical condition prior to practicing, changing your diet or consuming any nutritional supplements.

This book may include inaccuracies or typographical errors. The information is not guaranteed to be correct, complete, or up - to - date but is put forth in a best effort manner. All pictures have been edited to provide a more detailed view. Chairs and other objects have been removed. We promise better quality pictures as we become better editors and are very supportive and thankful to open source software and our favorite Gimp.

Tai Chi Chuan

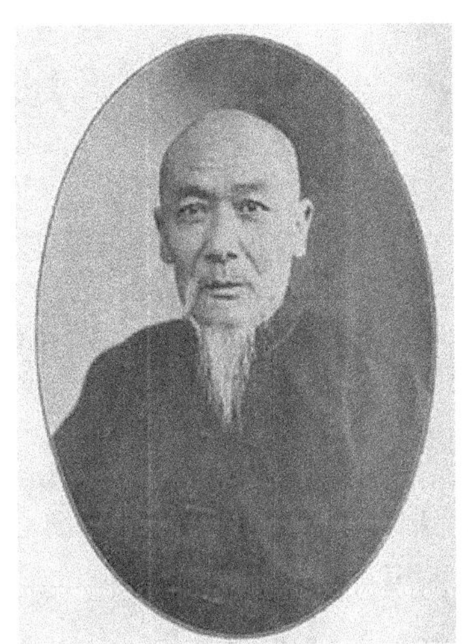

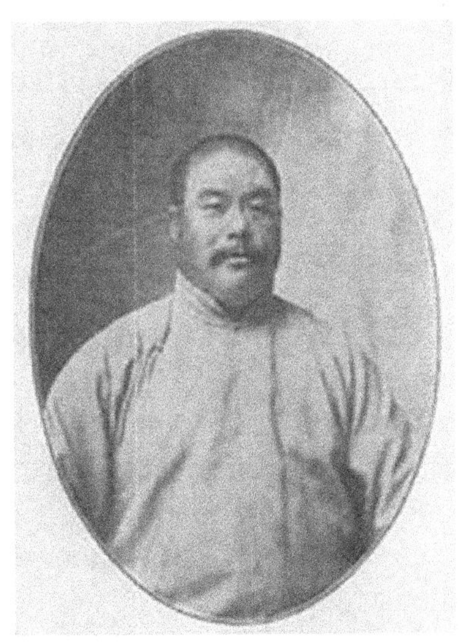

The Tai Chi Chuan Form

Tai Chi Chuan is an ancient martial art that has evolved into a healthy exercise. Tai Chi Chuan is one of the three major internal martial arts birthed in China – the other two being Bagua and Hsing I. Tai Chi Chuan, being the softest of the three arts, has become the most popular and can be practiced by all individuals. There are many varieties of Tai Chi Chuan. The most common being the Yang, the Chen and the Wu styles. The Yang system, which is the most popular of these styles, is often taught with the emphasis on health improvement, as is the lesser-known Wu Style.

People who regularly practice Tai Chi Chuan have general health improvements and develop better balance. Tai Chi Chuan practice has been found to help in the management of many other health issues. Common ailments such as arthritis and high blood pressure show marked improvements. There is much research being conducted into the benefits of Tai Chi Chuan using scientific measurements. The masters of the art know that Tai Chi Chuan benefits the whole body and allows the body to heal itself. Not all conditions are capable of being healed but a healthy body is better able to deal with its diseases when kept at its best.

Tai Chi Chuan is an art that has many facets to it. Anyone studying the art can spend a large amount of time training in all of its many facets – from bare-handed sets, two person sets and the many weapon sets. Beyond which there is the study of the impact of Tai Chi Chuan on the body, the meditative components and the esoteric theories involving yin and yang and five-element theory. This volume will touch on many of these components but will cover the most commonly taught principles and practices.

The form often taught as Tai Chi, is only a portion of the art of Tai Chi Chuan. Tai Chi Chuan is a complete martial art that also has incredible health benefits that have made the form popular with millions of people. Unfortunately, there are only a few true masters of the art, they are growing old, and many have passed. We need to work as hard as possible to get their knowledge and wisdom of the art. This book is an understanding of that taught by a select few of these masters

Tai Chi Chuan is not easily taught in a book. A book is a good resource to get deeper knowledge. As Grandmaster Liang used to say, you have to have teachers and you have to have books. He sat in his soft chair with a book on some part of the Tai Chi Chuan art, most likely an exotic sword form, working out the details on the form in his head or with a student. Between classes, William Chen is seen at his computer looking up some information on the body so he can explain to his students more about what he does in his art.

This book will try to follow a pattern but will be more a series of lessons focused on a specific part of the art. It is easier to look at individual aspects and explain about that portion of the art than to try to discuss a larger part with its many nuances. When possible a topic that has complexities will be discussed with terms that may need further explanation. This will allow the topic to be covered and the separate items discussed later. This is something whether it is about martial arts or atomic theory – it needs to be broken down.

Form

The Form is simply a series of movements put together to create a routine that can be easily remembered. Creating a form was done to allow easier learning of the movements. Many people were illiterate or books were expensive in the early days of the martial arts. A teacher may have written notes but publishing was not within their realm and the way of passing on the knowledge was to teach a movement and application that the student could learn. Originally, the art was taught one movement at a time until the student had mastered that movement and its nuances. When the art was taught more openly and to more students, it was more practical to teach a series of moves that could be practiced together. From this came forms in their many varieties.

Originally, the Yang form was a long form of 100 plus movements. The Professor who learned the long form originally taught it but in his estimation and maybe impatience, shortened the form down to what he considered the basic movements. The Professor's form is now generally known as the 37 movements although counting the repetitions it comes out with 61. Interestingly, Grandmaster Chen teaches his 60-movement form that is almost the same as the Professor's form with the exception of some additional movements. We are also seeing the development of other new sets taken from the basic movements of the long form to create Yang sets of different numbers of movements - all being subsets of the original form. Included lists of various forms in this volume cover the long form, the Professor's, Grandmaster Liang's and Grandmaster Chen's forms as well as many of the newer short forms.

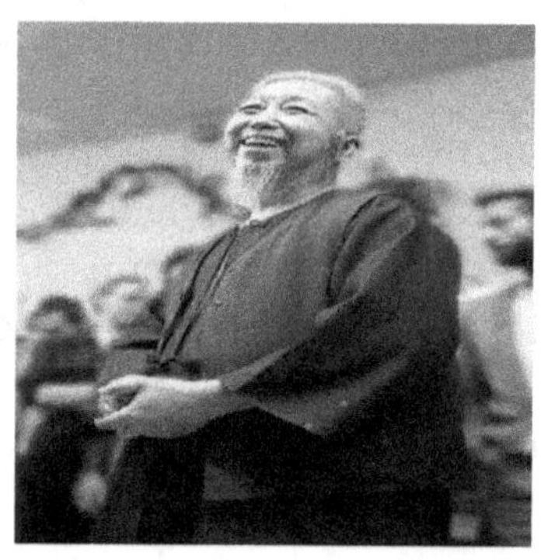

The long form was taught by Grandmaster Liang and the long form is still taught by Grandmaster Chen. Grandmaster Liang thought that the long form was required to move the Ch'i[2]. He recommended doing the long form right side, left side and then the right side again to get the full benefits of the form and moving the Ch'i.

The shorter forms have become popular due to the time constraints of the player's today. Teaching the short form definitely provides the largest number of students completing the form and with that completion, the student has a sense of accomplishment. Grandmaster Liang had said that the way to teach the art was to teach the form. Once the form was learned, the player would learn the left side of the form. Then they should start the dance - his 178 movements two person set. Only then should they be allowed to start weapon sets with the knife first and then the sword. He never considered teaching the staff and the spear while in Boston. Although he said this was the way to learn the art, he was very Taoist about it and allowed people to be in a number of classes with people playing Tui Shou before they finished the form and other players in various weapon sets.

Learning the form

Learning the form is the basic exposure to Tai Ch'i Chuan. After starting the form the fundamentals are required to advance in the art. This volume covers the majority of ideas that provide the basic background to understand not just the movements of the form but why and how to do them. Continuing with this series of volumes will provide a valuable foundation in the art.

Playing the form

It does not matter what version of the form a player knows but they start learning the first day and complete the learning process the day they die. This is a lifelong art. Practice every day and study more than just the form to understand Tai Chi Chuan. Develop a schedule so that there is time to play in the morning and in the evening. Then remember the whole form is not necessary for practice. A few minutes can be used to practice a part of the art. Waiting in line practice weight shifts and steps and no one will be the wiser.

Books, magazines, and videos are good for study but to get any serious information, a teacher is needed to study – actually many teachers. Grandmaster Liang talked of 17 teachers. Grandmaster Chen studied with the Professor as his main teacher but he also went to other sources to study related techniques even attending a boxing gym. Every teacher brings to their art their own flavor. Consider the study of the martial arts as creating a pyramid with many teachers at the bottom giving a strong base and then with progress, focus study on the teacher that meets needs and expectations.

If you are new to the art, it is acceptable to start your study at any one of the local classes. Ask questions about the teacher's background and who have been their teachers and why are they teaching. Some people start teaching before they have even finished learning the form themselves. This will set you back and waste time and money. Your teacher does not have to be a Grand Master but it helps. Never pass up the chance to study with the best. Also look for workshops in your area. Many teachers have workshops that are open to anyone although some require you at least have an understanding of a form. You can broaden your knowledge of the art since most teachers put a lot of effort into a workshop. When conducting a week intensive in NYC, Grandmaster Chen would stay at his studio to keep complete focus on what we wanted to teach his students.

Once you start the form practice follow the teacher's every move.

The William C.C. Chen Yang short form of Tai Chi Chuan consists of 60 postures that are linked together to create a form. Some of these postures are repeated since they are used to connect sections of the form together. The postures are easily learned with repetition and following the group during practice. One benefit of participating in a Tai Chi Class is the group comradely that comes from practicing together.

Many times people look at someone doing the form and they say they can never do it since it is so hard to remember. Group practice eliminates this as an obstacle since it is easy to follow a group and where one stumbles someone else knows that part. If you watch the videos from China, people in the park are practicing usually with a leader who they all follow.

People wonder how long it takes to learn Tai Chi. The short form can be taught in 6 months to 1 year depending on the individual. Once the form is learned then the next level is refinement – there are so many things to learn in Tai Chi Chuan that it takes a lifetime of study. Once a player starts the journey and can continue studying and practicing for the rest of their life. As Grandmaster Liang said:" you will never be bored if you play Tai Chi". Even late in life when he was considered a Grand Master he was still studying.

Playing the Tai Chi Form

Many people do Tai Chi but only a few do Tai Chi Chuan. This does not require competition in Push Hands or Sparring. Just that the whole art is so much more than mimicking a form or two.

When talking about the Tai Chi Chuan form, players will say, they are doing or performing but the Chinese talk about playing the form. Consider the difference. Play to continue doing it all your life. Make it fun and experiment.

Each day play the form morning and night. The short form can be done in under 10 minutes. After time then begin to add the second side. A standard is to do right, left and right on a regular basis. With the pace of modern life, it is hard to make the time but at least once a week set aside the time to play the "three-sided form".

While developing the form also learn some basic Qigong and Daoyin exercises to broaden the base of your art. These techniques are as much a part of Tai Chi Chuan as is the form.

With advancement, there are other sets to learn. The Da Lu's are a series that involves two people and is quite popular. After learning a few sets or maybe the complete dance, advance to various weapon sets. The order is varied but most masters teach the knife and sword. Tradition is that these extended tools are taught in this order - Knife (Dao), Sword, Staff, and Spear. More information is in the Golden Flower series of Internal Arts books.

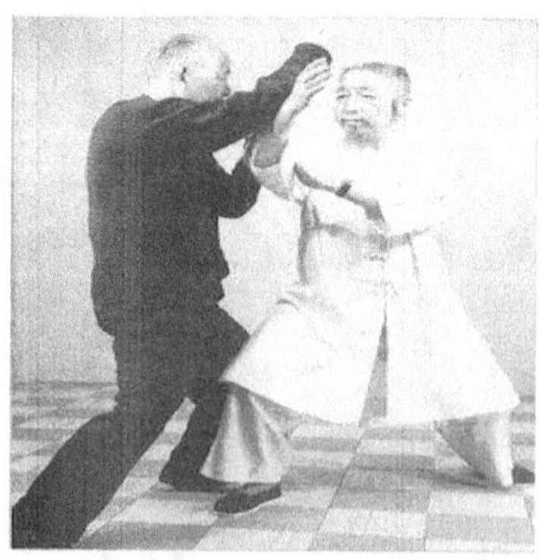

Anatomy

It is important to understand the anatomy of the body. This provides an understanding of the advanced theories of the art. Below is a high-level discussion of the body with a focus on the parts are of most importance to the Internal Arts study.

Foot

The foot is made up of 26 bones many without a joint, as we know it. These are actual joints since there is the capability of movement between the bones as they are attached bone to bone with cartilage. This provides flexibility in the foot when it is relaxed yet gives a strong stable structure when the weight is set. The foot takes the pressure on the outside edge (most of the time) and then as the weight is transferred into the arch of the

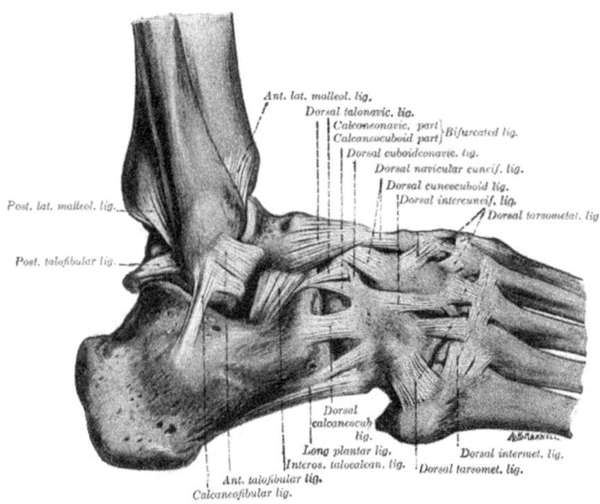

foot the bones lock into place providing a secure platform with the weight transfers. This allows the energy to be expressed from and through the foot.

The capability of the foot is severely limited due to our tendency to pack it into too tight of a container (too tight shoes). If the foot is allowed to function as it is designed, the flexibility is impressive and adds to its functionality. The foot can be trained to be flexible enough to pick up objects. It consists of a number of joints that can regain flexibility with proper exercise.

• The foot is the start and end for a large number of meridians.

• The foot has the flexibility that works with the inner ear and eye to keep us in an upright balanced position.

• The toes can be flexible enough to aide in the holding of a surface i.e. the grabbing into sand or earth to power the body.

• The foot has movement in 4 directions

• Foot has tissue that acts as a sponge absorbing blood and then pushing out with the weight transfer.

• Arch is flexible.

Bones of the foot, even when connected in an unmovable joint, have flexibility which allows the foot to flex and absorb shock when walking running or jumping. All the bones lock when the weight is located on the correct spot providing a strong base.

Ankle

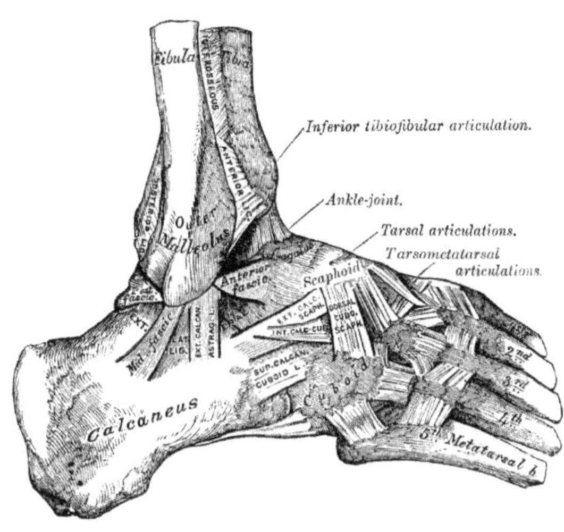

The ankle joint is usually less flexible than it should be. Efforts must be made to open this joint and get motion into it. From our walking and standing, we frequently allow it to become a stagnant joint that is used for stability while actually not providing the kind of stability that it was designed for. Beneath the true ankle joint is the second part of the ankle, the subtalar joint, which consists of the talus on top and calcaneus on the bottom. The subtalar joint allows side-to-side motion of the foot.

This joint is classified as a hinge joint. Hinges are meant to travel in one plane. Woodworkers and craftsmen are familiar with the design of the ankle joint. They use similar construction, called a Mortise and Tenon, to create stable structures. They routinely use it to make strong and sturdy items, such as furniture and buildings. This joint has more motion though allowing side to side motion but to a limited extent. Usually, this results in problems when it is overemphasized like in pronation. Remember that the motion best emphasized from the ankle is a parallel direction with the forward motion of the body Sprains occur when the ligaments are stretched more than normal. This results in a partial tear or complete tear of the ligament. This ligament damage results in the development of abnormal motion at the joint due to the loss of stability. When the back foot is out at a 45-degree angle, the foot still should be in alignment with the leg. The hip joint is the movable joint that allows this set up. The ankle joint needs to be worked daily to get the greatest benefit from the Tai Chi Chuan exercise and to provide the best balance as well as associated health benefits. Exercises for this joint can be done with or without weight bearing. The ankle can withstand 1.5 times the body's weight when walking and up to eight times when running.

Inside the joint, the bones are covered with a slick material called articular cartilage. Articular cartilage is the material that allows the bones to move smoothly against one another in the joints of the body. Remember that this material is constantly being replaced. Regular consumption of Break Bone Soup[2] now known as Bone Broth Soup will provide the needed material for repair and maintenance.

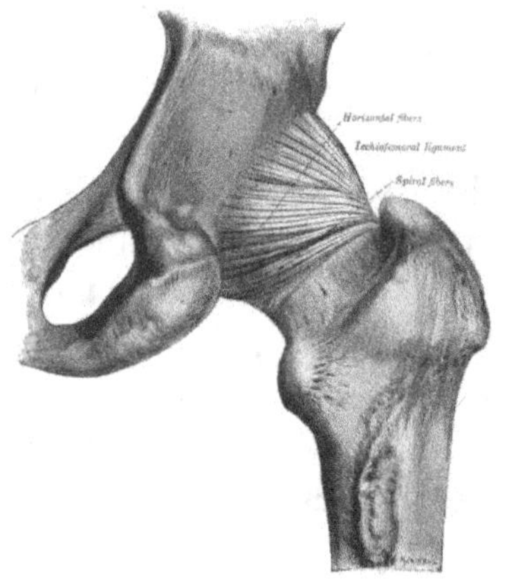

Hip

The hip is a ball joint allowing movement in all directions. Being a ball joint, it is supported by strong muscle sheaths to prevent excess movement and prevent the popping of the ball from the joint. Both flexibility and strength are required to keep the joint healthy. It is important to move the joint in as wide a range as possible to keep the joint socket lubricated. Excess use in only limited or directional movements leads to deterioration making this one of the commonly replaced joints in the body.

Excess stretching places stress on the ligaments and can overstretch the muscles leading to instability.

The hip is a critical point in Tai Chi Chuan. It is one side of the pelvic girdle and provides the channel of movement and energy from the stance into the posture.

Shoulder

The shoulder is a major structural component of the body and of the form. The bone structure the arm and clavicle form an angle into the spine. If the shoulders are raised the clavicle is directed into the spine in a downward angle. This holds the spine down and prevents the separation of the vertebrae. When the shoulders are relaxed, the clavicle is moved away from the spine allowing the spine to raise and separate the vertebrae. The shoulders maintained slightly forward also allows the slight hollowing of the chest but this posture does not close up the pulmonary cavity but allows it to expand in a direction out to the side of the body. This allows for the diaphragm to expand and the lungs to fill up the added space with air and successfully increase the oxygen transfer and noxious gas expulsion.

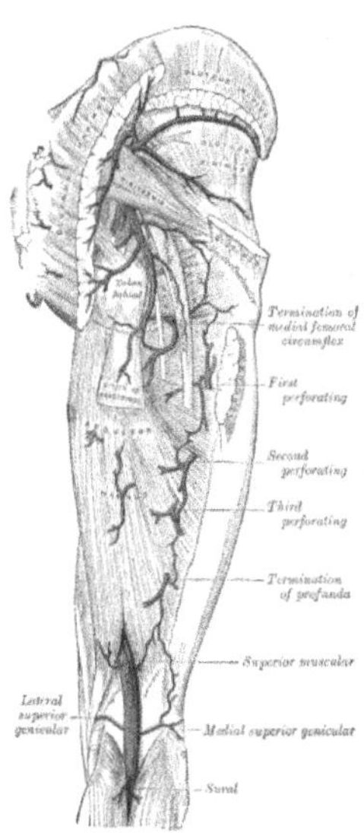

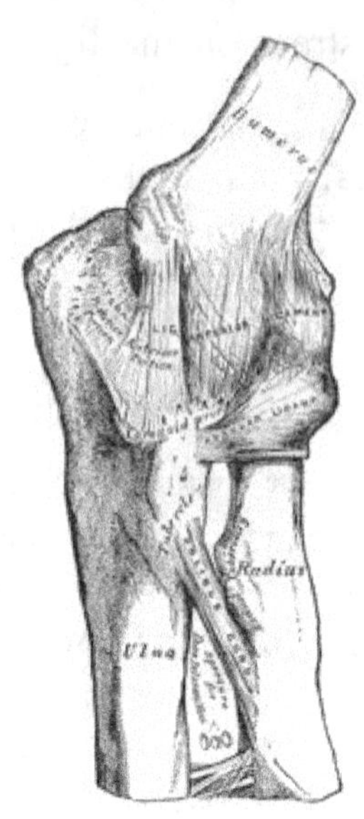

Elbow

The elbow is not kept down in the form. It is relaxed and moved outward from the body that actually raises it slightly. This movement along with the relaxing of the shoulders allows the rib cage to expand. If the elbows are pressed to the sides, the rib cage that is quite flexible is pressured into the body center. When the elbows are opened – think of opening the armpits or the arm Kua – the chest cavity is allowed to expand without pressure from the arms and increases the gas transfers in the lungs. The opening of the arm Kua also allows for the flow of energy out to the arms and the return of waste to the body. This is due to the opening of the Kua and allowing the transport vessels[3] to move the fluids with less pressure.

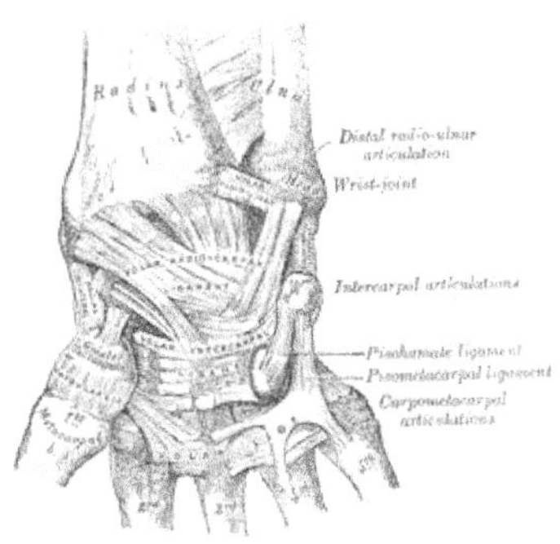

Wrist

The professor talked of the maintaining Fair Lady's wrist throughout the form. This was to allow the flow of energy into the fingers and back into the body. When the wrist is bent the pressure increases due to the kinking of the vessels and reduces the flow into the hands and fingers. Fair Lady's wrist for those who are not familiar with it, is to maintain a wrist that is not bent and the fingers are straight out and relaxed.

Back

Much is said about the back or more accurately the spine in Tai Chi literature. The emphasis is not misdirected. The spine conducts the power as well as the energy in the body. Whether a martial artist or practicing for health, the spine must be observed and corrected to get the full benefits from Tai Chi Chuan. When looking at the spine the first thing to know is that it should not be straight. There are natural curves to the spine that need to be examined. The bends must be evaluated to determine how close to a normal bend they are and how much correction is possible.

Starting at the base of the spine there is are fused vertebrae that form the coccyx and begin the inward bend of the lumbar vertebra. The spine then reverses to form the thoracic bend that goes outward from the body. The bend then goes inward connecting the cervical vertebrae to the base of the skull. This is frequently referred to as an S curve.

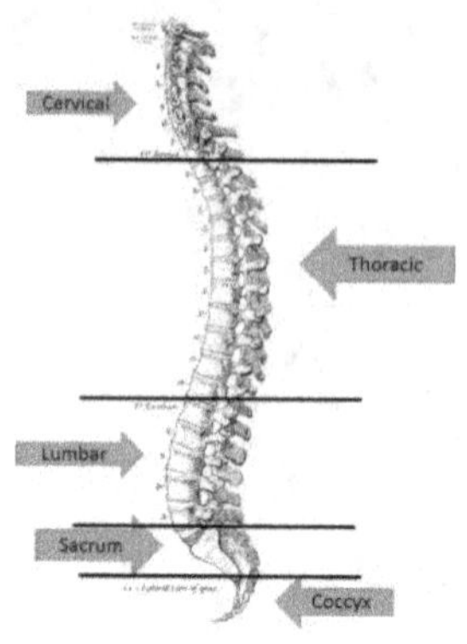

The bends all vary with the individual due to heredity and lifestyle. Some people are born with spines too straight that have very little bend. Others working at tasks during the day such as at a PC, develop an increased bend in the upper back.

One of the best ways to determine and teach what should be a student's best position is to use a staff or other long pole. Have the student stand in an upright position hold the staff at the side of the body. Basically, the head should be in line at the top and the hips should line up in the middle. Adjustments to bring these points in the body can be made by adjusting the weight on the feet whether it is centered, forward, or back. The hips may be thrown out of position. The head can be tilting forward. Shoulders can be slumped too far forward. All these issues can be pointed out and adjusted slightly. It is a long process to overcome these misalignments but recognizing them and subsequent adjustment can bring the spine into a position that will improve the posture not only in the form but in daily life which will lead to a better state of health.

Vertebra

Any work on the spine must be associated with an understanding of the vertebra. The human spine has 33 vertebrae 24 are movable vertebrae and nine are fused, five fused in the sacrum and four in the coccyx. The movable vertebrate has six minor muscles for adjustment and a cartilaginous disc separating them from each other. For visualization purposes imagine a rectangle with a muscle at each corner and one on the two long sides. Remember a muscles actions – it can contract to exert a pulling motion, it can hold using a number of muscle cells continuously firing until exhausted or it can relax allowing the muscle cells to lengthen. This process is being used to hold the vertebrae in place. These muscles are of a minor class as compared to the mass muscles of the body. Their job is to assist in keeping the spine in alignment so that it is able to react when the mass muscles require movement. Each of these muscles reacts to cause movement in the vertebrae to keep it centered on the disk and in line with the spine. Often we get issues when one of these muscles spasms and continues to pull or at least not relax. This can create issues with the

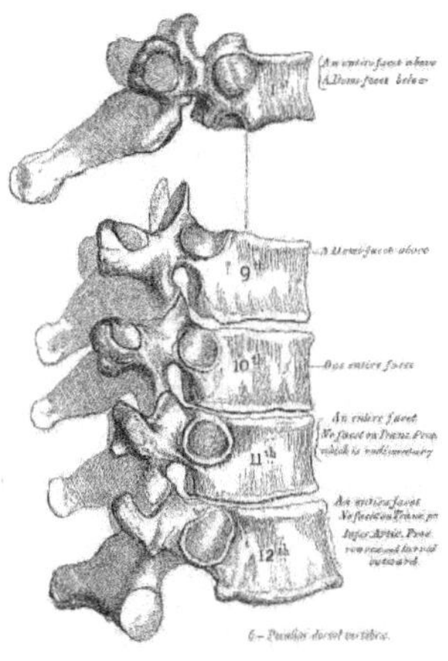

vertebrae being out of place and when movement is required, it can cause pressure on the nerves passing through it.

There are three nervous systems in the body, the Autonomic, the sympathetic and the parasympathetic. We control the sympathetic with our daily muscle movements. The parasympathetic and the autonomic systems are usually not under our control and function, as they are required for the body needs. With work, we can eventually get control of some of the autonomic and parasympathetic systems. One that is quite doable is the parasympathetic control of the minor muscles of the vertebrae.

Daily training in Tai Chi Chuan or its associated exercises can develop the control of the minor muscles of the vertebrae. The spine is mentioned frequently in the Tai Chi Chuan classics. The practice of Tai Chi Chuan will increase the flexibility of the spine and continued work will allow for more control of each vertebra. The simple expansion the spine when completing a movement will start the player in control of the spine. Working with exercises such as Phoenix rises from the ashes, bend the bow or the spinal bend[4] increase the connection into these muscles. Once there is a mental as well as a physical connection, the body begins to be healthier due to the spinal influences on the body. Every connection from the brain passes through the spinal cord and goes to the various organs. Examine the associated chart to understand what area of the spine affects which organ. Use this information to improve health as well as the form. In the William Chen system, the spinal bend is associated with every move. The relaxation prior to the initiation of the movement is a minor spinal bend where the spine is relaxed but the spine is maintained in an aligned position and upon the application of power; the spine opens and expands to allow the power to flow through it. Find out more about this in the other volumes of this series.

KUA

This is a mysterious name for a body part that does not exist. The Kua is the fold in the connection of the body between the leg and the thorax. This has a specific muscle structure to be discussed later. The Kua is either open or closed. There are two in the body. Actually, there are many more but we are discussing the major Kua of the body. The Kua closes when the body bends in half. In the west, we talk of bending at the waist. This is frequently done and results in many back injuries. The spine can bend which allow the bending of the waist but that is not an area that can take a lot of pressure. What is actually bending is a series of vertebrae that have limited range but add up to a bend. This is a good activity for health but not good for physical activity. When practicing Tai Chi Chuan, the Kua are used and the waist is not. The energy is connected to the root through the Kua and waist is not used. The back can be used as one of the bows of the body but this is an adjunct to the effort expressed by the body using the Kua connection of legs and thorax. The Kua is expressed in one of three manners.

- Single Kua open – single Kua closed

- Both Kua closed

- Both Kua open

You control the opening and closing by the bending of the body (thorax).

The Body

The organs of the body can be sorted into two groups for understanding their functions – the feeder organs and the processor organs.

Feeder organs do just that – they feed the body while at the same time they may also discharge the wastes accumulated from the bodily functions. These organs are listed below.

Feeder Organs

Lungs – Provide oxygen and remove waste gases from the bloodstream

Intestines – provide the nourishment from the food and water

Skin – a lessor feeder and more a waste remover but think of vitamin D created in the skin and the sweat and associated salts that are expelled from the body.

Processor organs have internal functions that keep the body functioning in an efficient manner. These organs are listed below. Not all of their functionality is listed below but the idea of their functionality is noted.

Processor Organs

Spleen – produces red blood cells

Pancreas – provides insulin for sugar balance

Liver- cleanses the blood of chemical toxins

Stomach – processes the food and provides chemicals to help the digestive process. There is some absorption in the stomach but the majority is in the intestines

Kidneys – remove waste products and excessive salts from the blood.

Bone Marrow – provides blood cells

Heart

The heart should be considered the conductor of the orchestra. It takes the blood in its expended state and sends it to the lungs to release waste gases and absorb oxygen. The heart then directly takes back the blood and directs it to all the organs to allow them to feed and provide nourishment to the rest of the body and release their waste products into the blood that is returned to the heart through the veins.

The Blood Vessels

There are three major categories - arteries, veins, and capillaries. Arteries control the blood pressure. The heat pumps the blood but muscles associated with the arteries narrow or expand to increase the pressure in the bloodstream. These are controlled by the parasympathetic nervous system - the one that controls itself. We have to realize that we do have control of our blood pressure when we can reduce our pressure through relaxation exercises and reduced stress. The veins bring the blood back to the heart to remove the waste products and gases and obtain oxygen and food products for the body. They use a combination of one-way valves and muscle contractions to get the blood back to the heart. These valves allow the blood to go towards the heart only. The pressure of the blood in the arteries is not enough to draw the blood out of the capillaries and push it back to the heart. The muscle contractions compress the veins and make the muscles into pumps while the valves prevent any back flow of blood. The capillaries allow the blood to reach the cells where the discharge of noxious gases and waste products and the intake of Oxygen and food products takes place with the blood.

Traditional Chinese Medicine considers that each organ has its own energy. The organs are separated from each other by a mucous membrane that surrounds each organ. When the body is in its proper shape the organs hang down and never touch each other. When they do touch the mucous protects them from the other. Over a period of time, if separation is not maintained the mucous membrane is reduced and the energy of the organs touch each other causing a poisoning effect that leads to poor function or malfunction of the organ and potential disease and sickness. This happens due to poor posture that we see in office workers or someone lounging in a chair too often.

Regular practice of Tai Chi Chuan can alleviate this issue and lead to increase the quality of function in the organs. The standard posture of Tai Chi Chuan is to maintain an erect spine sitting squarely on the pelvic girdle. The guidelines state to raise the head and straighten the spine while lowering the shoulder so the chest is slightly sunken. Raising the head helps to straighten the spine and separate the vertebrae. As the shoulders are relaxed, the scapula is moved away from the spine allowing for the spine to erect itself as the vertebrae separate. As the shoulders lower, the ribs are able to rise with the spine. This process allows the abdominal cavity to settle into the pelvic girdle – sinking the Tan Tien.[5] When the abdominal cavity is lowered the intestine and stomach are lowered allowing the remaining organs to separate and assume there proper hanging position. This also allows the diaphragm room to move downward. When a player takes an in breath it is the diaphragm tightening[6] which causes it to lower in the thoracic cavity and creating a vacuum in the pulmonary cavity. This allows the lungs to expand as the pressure open the alveoli and fills the lungs with air. The lungs, when remaining in a compressed cavity due to the limitations in the movement of the diaphragm when the body is in a compromised position, do not have the ability to fill completely. This allows the lower lung sections to maintain some air in the alveoli but not to discharge that air. As the blood flows into the lungs the air exchange takes place but the alveoli that are not functioning have a buildup of noxious gases.

This is alleviated when performing Tai Chi Chuan with the proper posture and following the breathing patterns. When in a proper Tai Chi Chuan posture the player takes in a full breath that fills up the lungs completely when the diaphragm can move downward unimpeded. This provides fresh air to all the alveoli. The controlled exhalation expels the waste gases and completely empties the lungs. We do this every day without realizing it. Our body needing to refresh itself causing us to yawn and sigh. Each of these actions allows for more complete exhalation of the lungs.

The normal breathing rhythm uses only the top third of the lungs in a breathing cycle. All the lower capacity is left until we exert ourselves or are forced to release the air through the yawn or sigh. When doing Tai Chi Chuan, we increase the amount of air exchange and provide for a more cleanse environment for the organs. The deep up and down movement also causes movement in all the organs allowing them to get increased blood supply and move to a proper hanging position. As a Traditional Chinese Medicine doctors said, the bell does not ring if it can't hang freely and so the organs cannot function correctly unless they are hanging correctly.

Ch'i Belly

There is a lot of good natured kidding about having a chi belly but often it is just a way of excusing extra weight in the abdominal region that is not good for the player's health. It is good to have some extra weight going into winter and then burn it off in the summer. That provides for warmth in the belly region, the location of the Tan Tien or triple heater. Also in the winter, more stress is on the body keeping warm and more people get sick. Having extra body stores provides for energy during a sickness. With age, it is harder to work off that winter insurance as the summer comes and it seems to stay with the body. It is a good idea to know what exactly constitutes a chi belly and what is excess weight. The chi belly comes from a number of reasons

Relaxation and development of the abdominal Muscles

Relaxation of the abdominal muscles allows for the development of space for the internal organs and the ability for those organs to assume their correct location. Breathing from the belly creates an expansion in the abdominal region. Just as in all aspects of Tai Ch'i Chuan, moderation is important. The increase of the regional needs to be monitored and controlled. The muscles of the abdominal region, the obliques, need to be worked correctly and monitored preventing excess fat development rather than relaxation for the development of the Ch'i belly. Limit your winter weight addition. Look at your body style and determine what a few percents of excess weight would be and set a date for that loss. Remember that as you age, the metabolism changes and removing weight is more difficult. Techniques of developing the abdominal muscles are in the next volume of Tai Ch'i Chuan.

Need to protect the triple heater

Wind can be a great risk to the body. Working out you should always protect the abdominal region from drafts. This can be simply wearing a t shirt in the summer or to wrap the region with a scarf in the winter. This is the area of the Ch'i storage and the warm needs to be protected. Tend the Rice Cooker.[7] As Ch'i stores in this region, protect it and nurture it as you would a puppy.

Additional body fat in that region

Age creates the possibility of less activity and the excess of body fat. Be aware of your index. Allow for some addition fat as a protective layer but manage it. Use the pinch an inch technique to allow for a layer of insurance and warmth but do not let it get too much. Understand that the body will develop a belly when the techniques of relaxation and breathing are followed but do not let it progress beyond that point. If you look at the pictures of the old masters you will see that even the thin ones have a Ch'i belly.

Playing Tai Chi Chuan

From day one, learn the techniques to improve balance. Walk in the most efficient manner that will improve the blood flow. Breathe to increase the oxygen in the blood but more importantly to remove to waste gases.

Playing the form without the Hands

The Professor once dreamed that he had no arms and had to play the form. The next day he said his improvement in the form was remarkable and all his fellow students noticed. It is essential to understand that the waist moves the arms and the hands. Otherwise, it is all hand business. One of the methods of learning the form that Grandmaster Chen teaches is to fold the hands in front of the waist and to do the form imaging that the body movements are taking place without the hands and arms moving. This reinforces the movement of the legs and body and takes the hand waving movements out of the practice. Subtle movements of the body need to be developed and are not lost in the large movements of the arms.

It is in the mind!

Tai Chi Chuan can be played by using the imagination and going through the form in the mind. Any part of Tai Chi Chuan such as punches and kicks can be practice in the mind. Having physically performed the movement it can then be performed in the mind. The engrams of the action will reinforce and will improve the performance of the movement. Many sports psychologists are using this as a training process. The Professor also talked about doing the same thing and many times just dreamed of doing the form. It adds up to more practice and an evaluation of the process of the movement in a more refined manner since the process can be done in slow motion and all aspects of the movement can be reviewed. When playing in Tui Shou[8] the player can imagine all the actions of each posture but not apply them to the opponent. This way punching and other techniques can be learned without risk to the partner.

Practice

Tai Chi Chuan must be practiced regularly to allow the Ch'i to develop within the body. Many people say they do or know Tai Chi but asked how often they practiced; many will refer to a class they took many years ago. Time, morning and night, must be set for basic practice and more time scheduled through the week for advancement. The Professor always said form morning and night. Doing the short form, a round does not take much time. Look to extend practice time a little at a time. Each minute of practice adds to the building of Ch'i and the extension of your life.

Development in Tai Ch'i Chuan is much more than playing a form. The list below contains just the basics to develop the practice of Tai Ch'i Chuan. Yang Cheng Fu writes of doing the form 17 times a day. Just learn all of these practices as they relate to Tai Ch'i Chuan and practice what you can when you can. Grandmaster Liang would say that he could never be bored since he started Tai Ch'i Chuan. There was something always to play with!

Solo form
Posture Practice
Punching and Kicking Practice
Daoyin
Qigong
Weapons
Weight Training
Running or walking
And More

The 13 Postures of Tai Chi:

The 13 Postures is the foundation of Tai Chi Chuan. Without the 13 Postures there is neither the Chuan (form) nor the push-hands. These 13 postures were derived from the Eight Trigrams (the first 8 postures - energies) and the Five Elements (the last 5 postures - steps). The 13 postures are:

The first eight postures are actions either defensive or offensive.

- Peng (ward-off)
- Lu (roll-back)
- Chi (press)
- An (push)
- Tsai (pull-down)
- Lieh (split)
- Chou (elbow strike)
- Kao (shoulder strike)

These five postures are actually movements allowing the previous postures to complete.

- Chin (advance)
- Tui (retreat)
- Ku (look left)
- Pan (look right)
- Ting (center)

A complete explanation of the 13 postures is in Volume 2 of the Tai Ch'i Chuan series.

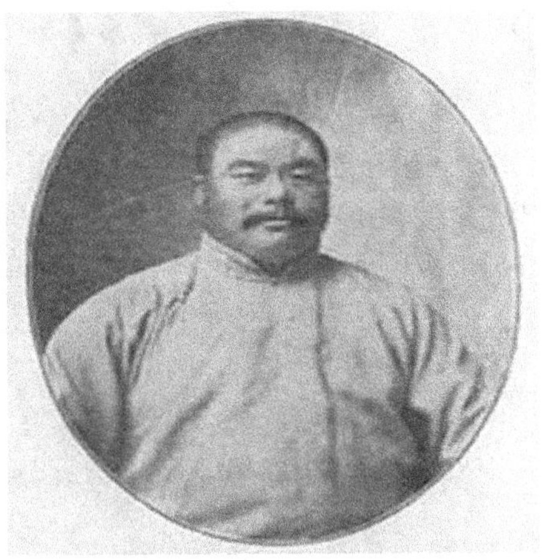

The 13 Principles of Tai Chi:

The 13 principles must execute the mind, chi, and physical movement in one unit. This means that when the mind is focused on a specific area of the body, the chi will flow into that area. When the chi flows into an area, power will follow. Each of these principles can become an entire volume. Each will have some discussion. For a complete review, the second volume of the Tai Chi series will delve into the internal work of this art.

1. The sinking of Shoulders and Dropping of Elbows

2. Relaxing of Chest and Rounding of Back

3. Sinking Chi down to Dan Tien

4. Lightly Pointing Up the Head

5. Relaxation of Waist and Hip

6. Differentiate Between Empty and Full: Yin and Yang

7. Coordination of Upper and Lower Parts of the Body

8. Using the Mind Instead of Force

9. Harmony between Internal and External

10. Connecting the Mind and the Chi

11. Find Stillness within Movement

12. Movement and Stillness Present at Once

13. Continuity and Evenness throughout the Form

A full discussion of these principles is covered in the 2nd volume of the Tai Chi Chuan series. A simple explanation to start the process is discussed below.

The sinking of Shoulders and Dropping of Elbows

Lowering of the shoulder and elbow structure allows the spine to raise and the joints to open for free flow of energy.

Relaxing of Chest and Rounding of Back

The chest is depress which allows the back to release the shoulders as discussed above and the spine can then be free to open up and extend.

Sinking Chi down to Dan Tien

Sinking the Chi is the first step in promoting relaxation. The concentration in the lower torso relaxes the upper body muscles and the breathing deepens initiating a relaxation response.

Lightly Pointing Up the Head

Pointing up the head means the chin is pulled in allowing the head to sit straight on the spine. Since the head is very heavy any misplacement of the weight puts stress into the spine. Tucking in the chin also allows the neck to extend removing the crease at the back of the skull. This opens up the channels for energy flow and relaxation.

Relaxation of Waist and Hip

The waist in Chinese references the region of the torso at the hips. This is the area that bends naturally. Trying to bend the waist thinking of it as at the level of the navel puts stress into the back bone. Relaxing the hip joint and the muscular structure supporting the torso allows the upper body to sink into the pelvic girdle and connect to the supporting legs.

Differentiate Between Empty and Full: Yin and Yang

This warrants much discussion but here we will just point out that the player must use only the muscles necessary to keep the body functioning and performing the process necessary at that moment. A full muscle is yang and a relaxed muscle is empty.

Coordination of Upper and Lower Parts of the Body

Basic rule is whole body. Every movement is with the whole body and requires that the parts are moving in the proper order. Here Yang makes it simple. Have your feet under you when you walk or you will end up on the ground. Start there and find the movement in every action. The upper body requires that its action has a connection to the lower body and the root or its not internal work.

Using the Mind Instead of Force

An internal system requires that you work with the mind to understand each and every movement. You need the strength of hold the energy of each action. The mind will direct sufficient energy to the action with training. So, every movement should be visualized by the mind and not an action of muscular force,

Harmony between Internal and External

As above the mind directs and does not need to fight the body to complete an action. Practice with the thought that the mind is directing the body but understand that the body will tell the mind when something is not right. Let them talk and you will develop the harmony.

Connecting the Mind and the Chi

Chi flows naturally in the body. Do not try to change that activity. The body takes care of its requirements. The action of the body requires the movement of chi also. This is above and in addition to the natural movement. This is where the mind using the chi stored and controlled by continuous practice, adds to the flow of the chi to have the addition needed to complete the action. This is discussed completely in the second volume with a discussion of the types of Chi and there activity.

Find Stillness within Movement

Calm and collected. Each movement when playing the form needs to be slow and make it look pretty. This will exude the stillness. This is critical for development of the art for practical use. All action should not be broadcast ahead of time. Only after completion should the opponent know that the action has been completed.

Movement and Stillness Present at Once

The body is never without movement. At every moment there are movements internally and externally. The body continues to process the needs to stay alive. The body also uses micro movements to maintain it stance and balance. None of these movements are readily perceived. The body exudes an appearance of stillness.

Now if the body stays that way, nothing happens. The player stands motionless. The development of the concept of motion within stillness requires the understanding of the concept of moving the body from the original position to the position of action – the posture in the form. Rapid motion is a flag to the opponent. He will have time to react. Practice requires the stillness of the motionless to be added into the motioned. Every posture requires that parts of the body not required remain calm and still and only those parts requiring movement actual move but without flags to the opponent.

Continuity and Evenness throughout the Form

Following the above thoughts, they lead to the flow of the form. Tai Chi Chuan has been called water boxing and long boxing. Indicating the flow of water of the idea that each movement moves to the other without break. This is the power of Tai Ch'i Chuan. At any moment the body is balanced in its power through the movements not exhibiting breaks. An action in Tai Ch'i Chuan looks like any other part of the form. Just like the idea of drawing silk,[9] any break in the flow causes breaks in the flow of the Ch'i. As the chi flows it becomes stronger and more powerful. The art of playing the form is to develop the Ch'i. Just as a river needs to flow without dams, the playing of the form needs to maintain its movement in a slow and sustained manner. Much more on this and other energy issues in volume 2 of Tai Ch'i Chuan.

Yang's rules

We have been given a set of rules handed down from the Yang family on how to play Tai Chi Chuan. These are straight forward declarations. An understanding of the body allows the incorporation of the rules into our form and practice.

1. Keep the head upright as if suspended from above and keep straight

The head is attached to the body as a 20+-pound weight. It also houses the brain. We need to keep the head under control for two reasons. The first is that wherever the head goes the body goes. The second is the brain is needed to make all the decisions on movement. These simple statements are extremely important. The head needs to be upright so as the chin is not down and on the chest. This allows vision ahead and to the sides. As the Professor said, develop the 1000-yard stare. This gives a soft focus that allows greater vision of moving objects - like a fist. It also keeps the weight of the head supported on top of the spine and centered on the shoulders. This needs to be a soft but unyielding connection. If the head is struck, the body needs to move with the head to absorb the energy of the strike and prevent injury. When a blow comes to the head the head must move by way of the body. If only the head moves, any strike will risk injury to the neck. When the head moves alone, the vertebra will come out of alignment. The energy of the strike adds to the weight of the head. A large amount of torque affects each vertebra and risk injury to the spinal cord, the nerves coming out of the spine and / or the spinal disc.

2. Depress the chest and raise the back

The chest is the rib cage and the back is the scapulars. They come together into the spine. When the chest is pushed out, it raises the rib cage and closes the distance between it and the scapula. If the shoulders raise they make a wide V and the energy vector directs into the spine. This rule's intent is for the spine to raise which allows it to open up the space between the disks to allow the pressure to be relieved. This also straightens the spine - although retain the natural S curve - and the energy can flow up the spine. Depressing the chest allows the rib cage to separate and expand. The relaxation of the chest allows the upper region to relax and connect to the scapula. The shoulders move out and away from the body to complete this connection. The lower rib cage - the floating ribs - connects with the pelvic girdle to make a complete connection of the upper body to the lower body. This allows the spine to thrust upward just as the energy flows up the spine.

3. Loosen and relax the waist.

The waist in this instance is at the location of the hips. This is considered the area of the abdominal Kuas. The body must turn using the hips with the spine only following after. If the turn is at the mid abdomen, the vertebrae will turn out of alignment with the spine. Pressure applied at this time can cause damage to the discs and the spinal cord. The turning of the hip joints one opening and one closing, and maintaining the spine structure prevent injury and allow for the release of energy from the spine. Loosening the waist allows the rib cage to lower. The abdominal cavity sinks into the pelvic girdle allowing the organs to hang loosely. The muscles that support the pelvic girdle turn without effort. The "waist" allows the smooth flow of energy from the legs into the torso.

4. Distinguish between substantial and insubstantial

Substantial and insubstantial is the yin and yang. When the body is strong, it must be strong. When it must be weak, it must be weak. When the body must accept the incoming force, it needs to redirect that force. At even a higher level, the body needs to understand the degree of yin and yang in each of these actions. When expressing force, the whole body must be more yang than the opponent's force. Otherwise, the yang energy instead of going into the opponent will fill up the yin side of the body of the player. Tai Chi Chuan is the understanding of all the variations of yin and yang in every part of the form and when and how much it needs to be at any time. The use of yin is not weakness; it just appears to be to the opponent.

5. Sink and relax the shoulders and elbows

The shoulder represents the upper body and the elbows are the levers connected to them. When either is raised, it gives the opponent the ability to us that part of the body as a level to break the root. The shoulders allow the spine to move freely when they are relaxed. The energy can move up the spine and out to the arms through the shoulders. On a more esoteric level, the raising of elbows or shoulders puts a crimp into the flow of energy up the spine inhibiting the flow of Ch'i as seen in the diagram below.

6. Use the mind not force

Shen, Yi, Ch'i, Li is the mantra. Shen is the spirit, Yi is the mind, Ch'i is the energy, and Li is the physical energy. This is the path of developing an internal art. When using the mind, the energy is smoothly exerted but when using the muscles – li, the force is cumbersome. The mind can image the flow and allows for the generation of engrams that are specific firing commands for a movement. This allows the body to generate the energy from the root and use the muscles and joints from the feet to the hand to exert force. When muscles are directly activated, they contact and exert force in a generalized manner. This is wasted energy and puts the player[10] at risk of a counter of that energy since it is not focused at the opponent's weakness. This is where the mind boxing comes to play. We practice the form and imagine the possibilities of the movements. We practice the movements developing those possibilities and as we work through these stages, we are working the brain. To store these events, the brain creates engram[11]s - programming of brain's processes - to recreate the action. This allows us to detect the weakness we have planned for, call upon the associated engram, and exert energy. Since this is pre-programmed, the body reacts to the programming in the most efficient manner that has been drilled repeatedly and the mind can focus on the opponent rather than the process of generating energy.

7. Coordinate upper and lower body movements

Whole body moves but like a snake. The movement starts in the toes and moves up the body connecting each part together into a powerful flow of energy. The body needs to move like a geared machine. Each gear is connected to the next gear and as the gear moves the teeth interact moving the next gear. If the movement is not following the established order, the gears jam up. Try shifting a car without using the clutch or shifting to the wrong gear. Things go wrong. The body is the same way in internal arts. The energy comes from the root and has to flow through each muscle and joint to the point of expression. If the movements are not in order, the energy will stop and even hurt the player.

8. Coordinate internal and external movements.

What is an internal and what is an external movement? Unless we differentiate the two, we cannot progress let alone coordinate the two. Let us break down the difference between internal and external then we can easily see why these need to be coordinated.

Internal Movement

An Internal movement is a subtle change in the body structure that allows the body to adjust its position and the connections in the body in a manner that allows the most effective movement of energy through the body. What does that mean? The best explanation is to use an example. Relaxing one hip allows the other to take command of the energy flow. Another - relaxing the shoulder muscle allows the opening of the shoulder kua to allow energy to flow out to the arm. We learn all these concepts and practice them in each movement. The internal movements are subtle but make a large impact of the potential for energy flow.

External movement

An external movement is readily seen. It involves the movement of a body part to the position where it supports the energy flow. An example would be a step towards the opponent, a leg moving during a kick, or an arm movement during a punch. These are critical since they allow the connection to the opponent but are not the source of the internal energy.

Now it is easy to see why we have to coordinate internal and external. If the internal body is not set, the energy cannot flow. If the body has not moved to the opponent, we are not able to exert our force. This simple explanation is not as simple to perform. This is why we must practice using the mind to direct and get our internal alignments in place and then align externally and exert the force. This cannot be done in a smooth and powerful manner if it is not practiced until programmed into the mind and body.

9. Absolute continuation of movement

Movement is essential to keep the energy flowing. The energy of the body takes many shapes and forms. Even sitting the energy continues to move. The form creates a flow of energy adding to the normal flows and creating new energy flows. The energy used must stay fluid through movement or it will congeal. Just as in cooking, many things need constant stirring or the dish will be spoiled. Making gravy is an example. Stop stirring and it will lump. This is the same with the energy being generated by the form. The flow needs to be smooth and constant. Too fast and the flow may spill or overflow. The new paths[12] being used must slowly be opened and built up to take the energy flow. As the volume of energy gets greater with practice, the channels expand to manage the flow. If the form is not continuous, the energy will pool in areas. This can lead to serious issues. Energy that is not circulating can sour which leads to serious health issues.

The same concept of continuous movement is important from a martial perspective. Any gaps in the energy can be points of attack from the opponent. Stopping energy flow impedes the potential force that can be expressed when countering and attacking an opponent.

The gap between energy release and movement to the next position has to be infinitesimal since we are susceptible when the body is at rest.

10. Seek stillness in movement

How can you be still and still move? Note that it says seek. You can recognized the person that cannot keep up with whatever they are doing. You think that they need to calm done. Every time you play the form the mind has to be clear. The body has to act slowly but determined to get to its posture. It is like watching the surface of a large lake and you see no water moving when it is calm but you know that there is always movement in the water. You develop a watch for that energy in your body and your mind. The mind is always filled with monkeys wanting to go here and there. Let them run away as Grandmaster Liang would say. Let the mind relax but focus on what you are doing. That will give you stillness but let the body learn instinctively what each movement is so that they movement comes naturally without direction – only the focus on the image of the posture.

Rules, Rules and More Rules

Drawing Silk

Drawing silk is something not well known today but the process involves finding the end of the silk thread and unwrapping it from the cocoon. The slightest hesitations and continuation will stop the unraveling process and result in the silk breaking. This has become a significant image within Tai Chi Chuan study and practice. The smoothness of movement is essential to make the continuous flow of energy throughout the body. When moving in Tai Chi Chuan, the body moves as one unit and this has contributed to the naming of the art as long boxing for its continuous movement from one posture to the next without the aspect of stagnation

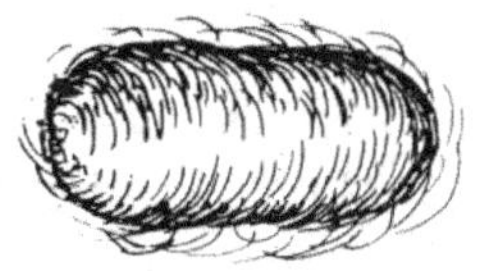

from a halting motion just as the process of yin and yang evolution passes through its stages.

Muscle Memory

Muscle memory is similar to a reflex action. Reflex action are designed in the body to do things like pull the hand away from the burner. A Muscle memory is a learned and repeated movement that the brain programs into its memory channels so the body reacts without conscious thought. Think of learning to drive. At first the brain is thinking off all the movements that are required to keep you on the road. After a while you never think about driving. Get in the car and go. The muscles and brain channels work without conscious thought unless required for a specific activity. Parking in your driveway does not need thought but parking in the space next to the high priced car brings the brain back into the equations.

Each movement in the form will become part of the muscle memories of the brain if practiced enough. This is not just to run through the form once a day. You need to work on each movement and understand it and repeat its motions until they are patterned in the brain.

Tony Knows

Who is Tony and what does he know? Tony's identity is toe, knee, and he has a nose. This is an important measure to detect the form's correct posture. When doing the form, be careful of over extensions – one of the most common is that of the knee. The knee can be extended too far forward or too far to either side and it will have a significant impact on the functionality of the knee. The knee is held in place by ligaments. The ligaments are the material that ties the bones together. Tendons tie the muscles to the bones. Stretch exercises are to stretch the muscles of the body – the tendons do not have much elasticity but the muscles get a stretching action from the individual muscle cells stretching or more accurately relaxing. The ligament is not a body attachment that stretches at all and if it does stretch, the result is very impacting. Once stretched a ligament does not return to its original shape. Ligaments that have stretched cause weakness in the joints since they become unstable and the bones of the joint can then travel outside of their normal range. The can result in complete breakage or tear of a ligament or a breaking of the synovial sac that encompasses the joint and provides it with lubrication. This synovial lining when torn causes leakage of the synovial fluid that cushions and lubricates the joint. When the fluid is not present and contained in the sac there is a grinding action. This grinding removes the bones protective coating and results in grinding of bone on bone all of which leads to arthritis and joint issues.

Therefore, what Tony knows is that the knee can be the most important connection in the body and it needs to stop at the toe. How do we test this? A common piece of wood - a broomstick or piece of strapping can be used. Place the bottom of the board at the front of the big toe. Move the body forward with the knee advancing until the knee touches the board. The nose should also only go to the position of the board so that there is a direct vertical line between the toe, the knee, and the nose. Also at the same time, check the knee's lateral position. There should be an inward incline of the knee. The knee when aligned strengthens its position and prevents the outward movement of the knee in the event of a push. This position will lock the body into the knee and then into the foot providing for the root and the power transfer without damage to the body.

The seven points discussed below are all related. These constitute the basic posture and stance of Tai Chi Chuan. Understand them and apply them to the body. Energy will flow through the body unimpeded.

Bend

Bend but Keep the spine straight

The spine bends to the left, bends to the right, bends backward and bends forwards. It can also be straight but the spine is never straight since its normal position is an S bend. When the spine is straight, the flow of energy is unimpeded. Any time upon initiation of an attack, the spine needs to be straight in not only a front and back state but also no tilt to either side. This aligns the vertebrae into a balanced state and prevents any kinks in the spine. Any misalignment results in loss of energy and potentially an injury from the torque when issuing energy. Neutralization is a different matter. A loose and flexible body and spine can segment when neutralizing an attack. This is risky since a hit on the body when segmented can cause injury. Training in neutralizing practices can allow the player to use, in some circumstances, a segmenting practice, neutralize the attack, and then use the energy of the assembling spine and body to launch an attack. Please read of this practice further in the document in the Tui Shou and San Shou sections.

Lower the elbows

The elbows move away from the torso. The release of the shoulders allows the elbows to move out from the torso. This action also allows the shoulders to lower. Combined these actions provide the opening of the armpits as described below.

Lower the shoulders

The shoulders relax and then move away from the spine. The lowering of the shoulders takes away pressure on the spine and allows the vertebrae to separate and the spine to raise.

Separate the rib cage

When the shoulders are dropped, the spine raises the rib cage. The upper rib cage, tightly attached to the spine, raises with the spine. The floating ribs lower, allowing a stretching of the thorax. This allows the pulmonary cavity to easily expand and collapse with the breathing process enhancing the gas exchange. The body's organs hang in their optimum positions.

Open the armpits – the Shoulder Kua

Do the bird

Grandmaster Chen refers to this opening as doing the bird. Think of the arms as the wings of a bird and the need for them to open out to get the bird in the air.

When doing the form, the joints need to be open – to allow for the flow of energy through them and to allow for the flexibility in a neutralization. The elbows do not exactly lower but go away from the body at a ninety-degree angle that allows the shoulders to lower and pull away from the spine. This creates a space between the arms and the body opening the armpits (Kua). It is thought to sink the elbows. This is the opposite of raising the elbows. The actual action should be to open the elbows. This is a movement away from the body. The elbows control the arms. The arm is attached to the shoulder and the shoulder is attached to the spine. Raising the elbows raises the shoulder that directs the scapula into the spine in a downward vector. This causes the spine to have pressure upon it in a downward direction causing compression of the spine. This compression of the spine inhibits the spine from functioning correctly. The spine needs to be able to pump the cerebral spinal fluid to the brain by its up and downward movement. The spine also needs openness to allow the nerves to have an unhindered connection to and from the other segments of the body.

When the elbows are down the body becomes closed. The arms move towards the body and close the Kua of the arm. This inhibits the flow of blood and nerve communication to and from the arm. The lymph node in the armpit (Kua) is under pressure from the arm. This limits the flow of lymph fluid through the body. Lymph fluid moves by alternating pressure and needs an uncompressed vessel to allow the free flow of the fluid. The rib cage is also restricted with the downward elbow position. The rib cage needs to rise and sink at the same time to join the body together as one unit. The fixed ribs raise and allow the organs to hang properly and the pulmonary cavity is expanded to allow for greater lung capacity. The floating ribs sink to allow for added organ room and a connection to the pelvic girdle.

If the focus of the elbows is away from the spine, the body can function at its highest ability. The elbows will open the Kua of the arm allowing full flow of the blood, lymph, and nerve communications. The scapula will move away from the spine allowing the spine to rise upwards. The rib cage will open up with the fixed ribs fitting into the gap created with the rising scapula and the lower ribs will sink to connect to the pelvic girdle. This creates a connection where the energy can go up the spine without hindrance and flow out the arms with the connection to the rib cage connecting to the pelvic girdle that connects to the base created by the stance.

The shoulder Kua - the armpit, opens to allow the energy to flow. Opening the Kua is done by the elbows. Think of the elbows as going away from the body to the sides. This not only allows the shoulders to lower but also opens the kua. The shoulders are then able to sit more squarely removing any hunched action on the body allowing the spine to rise.

Open the Joints

The joints of the body both the movable and the immobile must become flexible. The flexibility will aid in the body assuming the postures and to move fluidly between postures. Not only will energy flow smoothly through the joints but also the opened joints will allow for the unimpeded flow of the four fluids [13] of the body increasing health and vitality. Remember that the body joins bones together, IE. the foot and the skull where they are attached by cartilage and are considered immovable. These joints actually have an innate flexibility that can be increased with practice. It will make the body more flexible and able to pass energy through it.

Raise the spine

The spine is a finite level bone structure. How is it raised? The spine consists of some very important parts.

- Spinal Cord

- Vertebrae

- Discs

- Minor Muscles

All of these components are discussed in the anatomy section of this volume and are referenced in the Qigong and Daoyin volumes [14]. Control of these body parts allows management of the spine. The spine when raised is at its optimum posture. The alignment of all the components is correct. The spacing is correct. The spine tilts neither right of left. The spine tilts neither forward nor back. If all of these conditions are met, the head will sit on top of the spine. The head will not tilt in any direction. Looking at the player, the appearance is of height, straightness, and strength. Physically the spine is then in its greatest health. It functions to its ultimate capabilities. From an energy perspective, the flow of energy through the spine is unimpeded. The health of the player is at its greatest since all the energy can flow throughout the body. All this is possible when the spine is raised. All the components of the spine now function.

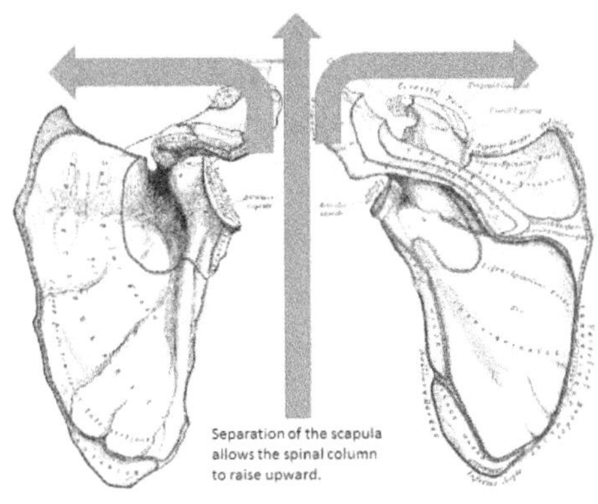

Maintain the head in an erect position

From an energy perspective, the head receives the energy going up through the back of the neck into the head and down the front of the face. If the head is bent forward, it cuts down the flow of the energy into the head. This also crimps the flow of the cerebral spinal fluid. The mind needs to be active and refreshed when doing the form. This requires the flow to the head[15] to go through a straight spine. Also having the head down, prevents correct focus and if hit in the head the torque from a bent neck can cause a rupture to the disks. A level head aids the balance since any inclination acts as a counter weight and throws the balance off. From the aggressor's perspective move the head and the body follows.

Maintain the Center

Tai Chi Chuan requires the principle of the spinning top. An attack is spun off to the side. The root is a single point to the ground. A two footed root is strong but limits the movement of the body where a single point of contact allows the body to spin and direct the attack away. The center is the rice burner. This part of the body exists in the pelvic girdle. The upper body and the lower body connect to the pelvic girdle. Movement of the upper part of the body, the torso, requires movement in the lower part of the body to counter balance the weight and maintain the pivot point. The perfect point of balance is with the torso directly over the root and the legs connecting to the single root. Neutralization and attack changes that position and requires the constant monitoring of the center. The body needs to compensate during the movements to maintain that center.

Open the pelvic girdle

The pelvic girdle is the bone structure made up from the hips and buttocks. It is quite flexible and is a major connection for the spine to the lower body. To get a connection, the pelvic girdle is relaxed which allows the coccyx to sink into the center of the girdle. To achieve this relaxation, the buttocks are separated and the hip muscles relax. This creates an opening of this region of the body. It also allows the abdominal cavity to

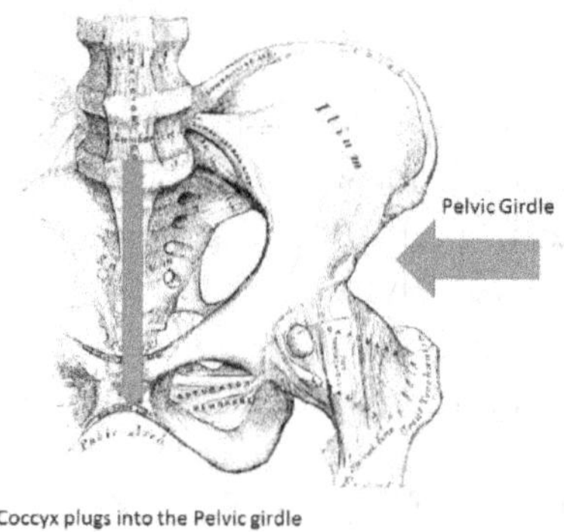

Coccyx plugs into the Pelvic girdle

sink downward freeing pressure on the pulmonary cavity and the internal organs.

Create the compression and do not lose the container

When energy is expressed, the body is yang. This is achieved by creating compression in the body. The compression comes from creating a container – the leg(s) and the shifting of the weight on to the leg(s). The legs become the container holding the compressed gas – think of it as an air tank holding compressed air. Upon the initiation of an action the value on the tank – the hip Kua opens and the air inflates the upper body creating the yang energy. Now thinking back to the tank, when the air is released from an air tank, the tank does not change shape. It is built out of steel shaped to hold the compressed air. The lower body is like the air tank and it holds the compression by maintaining the shape. When the gas is discharged, the lower body keeps the shape[16] – moving neither up nor down – only the upper body moves as the air (energy) inflates the body.

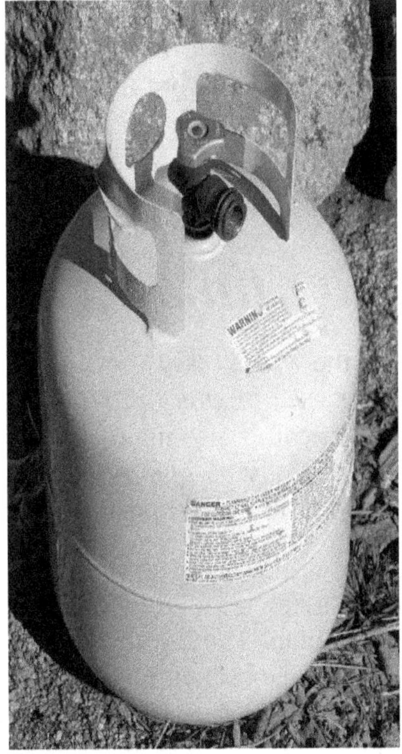

Compressed Gas

61

Compression

Compression provides the power in Tai Chi Chuan. It is likened to the power a tool gets from compressed air or hydraulic fluid. During the process of stepping into a stance and then shifting the weight to that foot, the body compresses energy into the stance. At that point, maintain the compression in the body. Imagine the lower body as a tank that holds the compressed air. When the tool needs power, the air is dispensed through a tube that powers the tool. The tank does not alter. If the stance rises with the dispensing of power, the imaginary tank changes shape. If it does change shape, the volume of the compressed air is allowed to expand and the pressure going to the tool or the posture is less. The stance must remain solid and compressed just as the tank does not change its form. Either the stance or the tank changing changes the volume and therefore allows the energy or air to have less pressure.

Whole body means whole body but all in due time

The whole body is not the movement of the whole body at one time. Tai Chi Chuan requires that the whole body be used in every movement. This is required for creating the power in a movement. It also maintains the balance of yin and yang in the form. The whole body as one movement such as a push where the step, weight shift, body turn, and push are all done as one movement is considered a clumsy movement.

If the whole body is used as one unit, there is no flow and the energy -it is hard and static just like the use of a club. The Tai Chi Chuan energy is the snapping of a bullwhip. At any time if the bullwhip is stopped in its movement, there is no impact. At the last moment, the bullwhip is connected to the root creating the snap of the whip – the energy into the opponent. The whip moved to its position but only through the movement of each section. The alternative is to throw the whip. Without it maintaining connection to root, it just impacts the target with the weight of the whip.

The principle of Whole Body starts with the root. The root is maintained at all times. The stance is created. The body then assumes a posture. When the action is taken, the energy flows just like in an electrical circuit - from the source – the root through the foot into the ankle, up the leg, through the pelvic girdle through the spine into the arm(s) into the hand and then applied to the opponent. At any time, the action is controlled and can be stopped. This is the softness of Tai Chi Chuan. That energy has moved through the whole body to provide the internal power of Tai Chi Chuan. It does take time and coordination to allow the flow to pass through each component in the body in their proper order.

Relax the jaw but do not leave the mouth open

Jaw muscles create and demonstrate tension. When we are tense, we clench our teeth. When we are under stress, we again clench our teeth with tight jaw muscles. The muscles need to be relaxed. This will help relieves stress but will also reduce the pressure on the nerves that pass through the jaw. The jaw cannot be too relaxed otherwise, the teeth come apart, and the jaw becomes slack. Upon a hit or even a hard movement in the form the slack jaw can be jarred. With a strike to the jaw the player may get a broken jaw. Less of a strike or a stumble when doing the form can send a shock up the nerves of the jaw that jars the brain.

The tongue is against the roof of the mouth

Keeping the tongue touching the roof of the mouth keeps it from being bitten upon a strike or a stumble. It also, more importantly, completes the energy circuit in the body connecting the energy flow from the head to the thorax. See the Inner Brocades volume for more information on this critical switch.

Breathe through the nose and release - let it go out both the mouth and nose as it wants to

Breathing in Tai Chi Chuan should be as close to natural as possible. For this reason, we use the post-natal breath and breathe in through the nose. The nose is the normal filtering process that also warms and moisturizes the air as we breathe in. Releasing the air allowing it to get out of the body whichever way is fastest and involves less effort. This allows the exhale to use both the mouth and the nose to exhale. This creates a larger pipe to get the air and its waste gases out of the body. Breathing in requires an effort of the muscles and the exhalation being as relaxed as possible, allows those muscles to return to their pre-expansion state. Relaxing and letting the air out provides for a quicker turnaround of the muscle state.

Even More Rules
Root

Just as a tree has roots the Tai Chi player must develop a root. The concept is the same as for a tree. The tree's root proves nourishment and connection to the ground. The Tai Chi Player's root provides nourishment of the Chi and stability of the body. Just as a deeply rooted tree does not topple the Tai Chi Chuan Player should have a deep root and not topple either.

Rooting is a complex process but the heart of the process is simple – the relaxation into the earth. Most of the effort in generating a root comes from the control of the mind. When the mind is calm and relaxed yet bright and aware the player can visualize the root and feel the earth. Once the

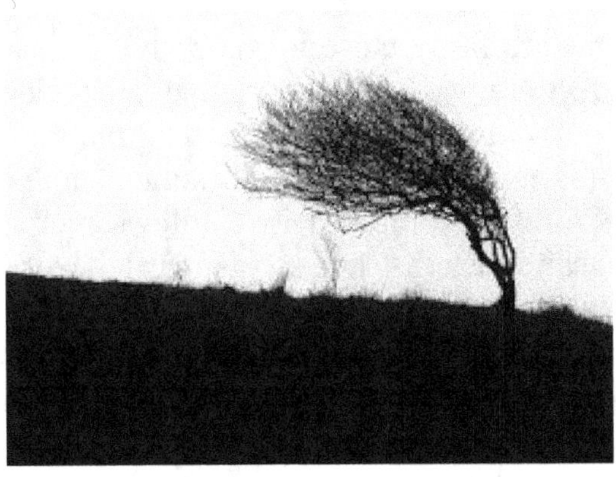

mind is in the proper state the player then practices techniques to allow the body to hold the root and prevent anyone from moving the player.

When discussing the root, here the focus is on a single weighted stance vs a double weighted stance. The stances are defined and discussed elsewhere. The root starts with the foot. The foot needs to be flexible and able to open and close the joints in the foot. When the weight is on the outside of the foot the foot is not stable and rooted. Once the weight is transferred to the inside of the foot the bones and joints of the foot lock and provide a solid foundation into the earth which gives the player the ability to establish a root.

When the root is established the body position always maintains a center over the weighted foot. The body is light and flexible but as it bends as in a willow, the weight is maintained over the foot by the movement of the hips knees and ankle.

This allows the player to bend far backwards in avoiding a push or punch but to maintain stability with movement of the three joints. This also allows for a quick response since there is no need to shift the weight before initiating an action.

Small Frame vs Large Frame

The Professor is credited with promoting the small frame Tai Ch'i Chuan. Small frame is when the feet are close together both in width and length and the arms are fairly close to the body. The large frame takes a stance where the feet are wide apart more than a shoulder's width and the feet are stretched out with the rear leg far behind the front foot. Simply the difference is that it is easier to do the small frame than the large frame – the main reason the Professor promoted it. It allows more people to do the form and get the health benefits. For all his martial expertise the Professor was foremost a doctor. Over the years students of the Professor has deviated from this teaching. Ben Lo has an extremely low and large frame. This does not make his teaching incorrect just harder to do his style. Grandmaster Liang was more a middle of the road stance. Grandmaster Chen has taken the teaching he received from the Professor and not only worked on it reduce it more but to emphasize the martial aspects of the compact stance. In the original Yang teachings, the large frame was taught first to develop expansion and muscular strength and as students advanced they would close up their forms and end at the small frame.

Fair Lady's Wrist

Fair Lady's Wrist is something the Professor insisted on in his form. It differs from the early Yang practice that uses a raised wrist in many of the movements. The reason for this change had to do with the understanding of relaxation and energy flow that the Professor was bringing to the practice of Tai Chi Chuan. Grandmaster Chen has taken this even further by studying the nerve enervation of the muscles to determine the proper hand and finger position to provide the relaxation as well and the greatest power in the movement.

Fair Lady's Wrist consists of the hand, wrist, and arm to be in direct alignment. This allows the wrist to remain relaxed and open. The movement of blood and lymph fluid is increased since the wrist joint is open and relaxed. This position also allows the fingers to be the controlling action in the movement. When the hand is in the raised position with bent wrist, the fingers lose their flexibility, the ability to activate the required muscles and to control the energy flow.

Four Corners

Four Corners is referenced to the cardinal directions when playing the form or as one of the pushing hands forms. This reference to four corners though, is to the body - the torso in particular. When looking at the torso, there are four corners of the body – the two hips and the two shoulders. The corners create the form that manages the power of the postures. The squareness of these points creates a solid structure. If one point is not in the same plane as the other points, the torque of any movement loses it support structure.

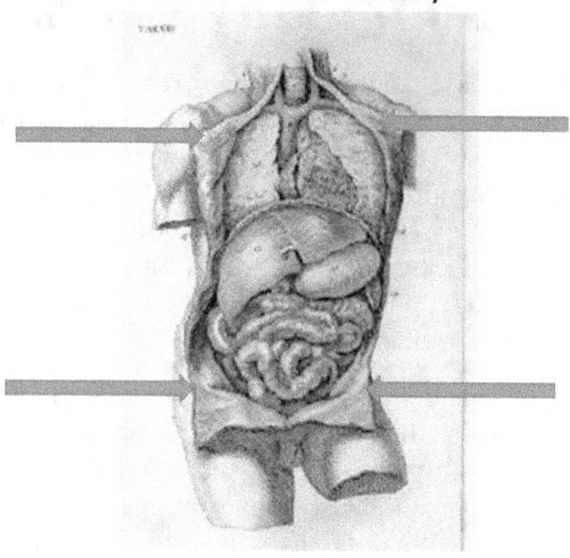

The shoulders are square and open in the same plane. The hips are also in the same plane. This creates the box as seen below. A box is strong and can disperse its load throughout. Tai Chi Chuan uses this concept moving energy up from the legs and into the torso. The upper body is balanced with Yang energy. A point out of alignment is less yang and thus the yang energy that is filling the torso will move to the yin point rather than be directed to the point of attack. This is a practice used throughout industry. It is known that back injuries are the cause of much loses in productivity. Directions for lifting objects stress the alignment of the body. This is a simple concept to understand. It must be incorporated into practice.

Neutralization in Tai Chi Chuan uses the concept of four corners. If an attack is to a shoulder, that shoulder will detach from the structure, becoming yin and moving with the energy applied by the opponent. The opponent's energy is dissipated into the yin shoulder. When the action is completed, the body realigns and the square attacks. This technique is demonstrated the Tui Shou volume. This is part of any quality push hands practice and it is a standard warm up exercise.

Another part of the four corners is that each of the corners is an energy hub. While playing Tai Chi Chuan, the advanced player feels the energy. Again, this is a topic of discussion in a later volume.

Four Corners

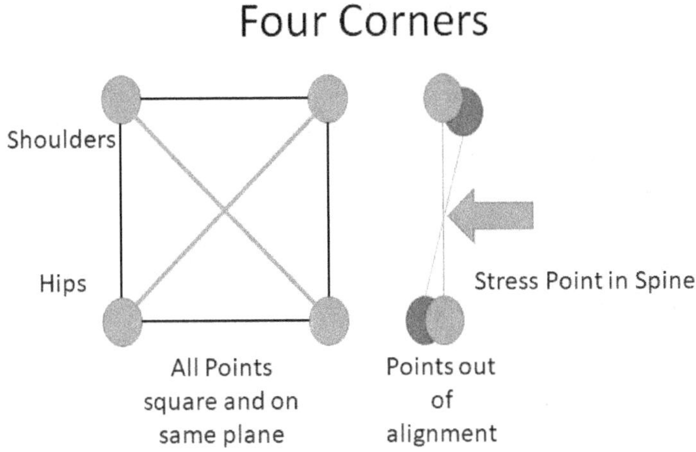

Do not Break the Back

This rule goes with the prior rule for principles in maintaining the proper posture to use efficiently project energy and to avoid injury. The back and hips, when maintaining the four corners, create a plane as seen in the diagram. This plane establishes a position where the hands stop. This maintains the power and structure of the torso. The joints work in the frontal position. Moving the hands further then the plane, puts the joints out of their proper position. Energy cannot flow smoothly. The joints are injured when in these positions.

Softness

Develop softness in the form. Only through softness, will the energy flow. Starting with softness evolve and create hardness when required. Softness can easily be brought to hardness but hardness is much more difficult to make soft. Energy flows not only up and out but also down and away with the body only being a conductor of the energy. Hardness in the path will cause congestion and not free flow of the energy. Think of a bullwhip. It works by using its flexibility to flow through the whip to its end. Put a link of metal in the middle and the motion will stop when it reaches the link.

Make the shape

The ending shape of the posture is more important than any shape getting to that point. Grandmaster Chen sets the player in the final posture. This creates an engram. The player then relaxes out of the posture and then assumes the proper posture again. This reinforces the engram. The player can learn all the small movements only after knowing what the shape looks like at the end of movement. This has proved very effective. The player learns the posture and can continue learning the form. Progress is made. The player makes the movement smoother as the numbers of repetitions are completed. The attitude of the student remains positive. The transition movements improve. Corrections are given in an assimilated manner.

Ending is just a thought

Form is the culmination of a series of movements that set up a completion in those movements that mimics an application in the martial tradition of Tai Chi Chuan. Many things go into making the movement of the body parts and the mental intent to comply to the traditional Tai Chi Chuan techniques. One area that is fraught with variations is the ending of the movement prior to proceeding to the next application. From the very beginning, there is the slightest hesitation between movements but there is often an emptiness in that moment. Grandmaster Chen puts clarity into the form by using his technique of go asleep and to wake up. The movements of setting up the body to complete the application are done in an unfocused state – not unaware but in total relaxation. This keeps the body in a state of yin energy that does not alert the opponent to the action and allows for an alteration of the action – neutralization most likely leading to either the completion of the intended movement or to evolve into another one. When the body is set the mind takes on a level of the awareness – awakens. This alters the yin to yang and gives the power capability to the movement but in the form it is only the thought of action.

Take a Pose

Grandmaster Chen also like the thought of taking a pose or a picture. Think of how you change your attitude when someone says they are going to take a picture. You empower yourself with energy and alertness. Being a student of Tai Chi Chuan, you do not stick your chest out and raise your shoulders but your head elevates and your shoulders sink yet your ribs raise up. Your energy is available. Using this image in the form for the ending of the movement enlivens the form and draws the yang energy into the body from the root.

Practice your form with your mind knowing that someone is photographing the ending of the movement. Once you start, continue for all movements in the form. You will begin to see the images that you need to complete in your mind and you will feel the energy moving into your body. Go out and take all the movements and practice them individually but set them up to end with the image in your mind that you are taking a picture of the movement and what you want it to look like. Continue this and you will note the great improvement in your form.

Remember when practicing the movements in a static position that the phrase burning it in can be taken two ways. One is to burn it in to the ground and ashes and the other is to burn it into flames. You want the image of flames to bring the energy up into the body rather than burn it down to ashes and into the ground. This is a simple mind image but you can see the difference when you practice and also with many people who talk of burning it in and their posture just keeps getting lower and more static and unable to move. Movement provides energy.

Check Yourself

The player gets in the habit of making movements that become habitual and programmed into the mind and body. When playing with the form or an application, stop and review the body and all the components. Are the alignments correct? Is the weight correctly balanced? Is the breathing correct for that movement? Are the movements in the correct manner? Is the movement directed by the mind? Only by stopping and evaluating the form, can the habitual movements and practices be evaluated. Remove those that make the form and the movements suffer and enhance those that improve the form.

Circles and Circles within Circles

Keep the limbs rounded. The joints need to be open and all the joints slightly bent. Not only does this help prevent locking holds on the joints but promotes the flow of energy and the body fluids. When the limbs are rounded, the movements can become part of a circle. Everything becomes a curve. The circles come from any direction and never end so each movement can flow into the next movement. At any time, the force vector can be initiated when the movement is circular. Just like a ball, everything can roll and spin off into another circle. The force may be coming up through the body and then roll to the side directed downward just as done in roll back. Keeping the limbs rounded allows the joint to open. When the joint is not locked, the tendons and ligaments maintain a level of flexibility that allows bones to move away and provides space within the joint. The synovial fluid resides in the joint capsule evenly distributed and lubricating the bones and cartilage allowing for a smooth and friction less movement of the joint. The helps prevent the development as well as heal arthritis.

Areas where joints are commonly locked can be in the arms in strikes and pull downs. In the knee in retreat such as roll back. All these places should be evaluated and corrected in the form.

No Waist Just Fingers and Toes

The actions of legs and waist are all the preliminary movements. The gun is loaded and all that is needed is to pull the trigger. This is the action of the toes initiating the release and the fingers directing the energy. If the body is not in a ready position, the energy is directed to the movement of the body to that position. This action grants power to the stance. The body movements, correct stance, and posture provide for the loading of the gun (body). The body is ready for the attack. The toes and the fingers release that energy (FA or AN Jin as described later). When the fingers and toes release the energy, the body may follow but is only the passage structure for the energy and not the source or director of that energy.

Toes and fingers are the only movements the rest of the body follows

When playing the form, the hands and the feet should be the point of focus. The hands must be connected to the body by the Fair Lady's Wrist but the hand itself should be relaxed during the motion until the end of the movement. The fingers can be slightly bent but the hand should not be closed. Upon reaching the end of the movement, the index and middle finger energize and the thumb directs the action.

The foot makes the connection to the ground where you gain your root that supports the energy of the movement. The foot is divided into three points – Grandmaster Chen's three nails. The toe is the action point (little brain) and activates to start the flow of energy from the root. The ball of the foot acts as the secondary root providing support and rooting actions. The second nail is used when expressing energy supporting the big toes when it activates. The third point is the heel. It acts as the stabilizing root. It provides a support to manage the energy from an aggressive attack. The heel also provides a rooting connection during the action in a movement when energy is not being expressed. More of this energy connection in volume 2.

Many people will think that the expression of energy such as a push or a strike is stronger when the foot is firmly planted on the heel. This is not so. The energy is expressed with the heel disconnected from the ground. It may be touching but by rooting on the heel, energy will only be held back. In this manner, the heel can act like a sailing anchor putting a drag on the body and preventing the complete expression of energy. In the same manner, the rear leg must be activated moving into the rooted leg and unattached or lightly attached to the ground to allow the free turning of the pelvic girdle.

To understand the importance of the hands and feet in Tai Chi

Chuan is to understand the balance of Yin and Yang and how they work in a martial art. Yin and Yang may be two opposites but the true understanding is that nothing can exist as pure Yang or pure Yin. There are varying degrees of Yin and Yang. Consider that something like one hand is more Yang than the other hand but in consideration to the opponent they must be both Yang hands for an attack. What makes them yang is that they are more Yang then the opponent when striking. This allows impact and energy to go into the opponent. If both hands and feet do not maintain a level of yang-ness higher than the opponent does, the energy expressed will travel to the less yang area - IE. your yin hand and not into the opponent. Whenever completing a movement, two hands and two feet are activated making them yang in varying degrees. This is to balance the body in relationship to the opponent who should be less yang and therefore receptive to the energy. Yes, Yin can beat a very yang opponent but that is a different discussion. Here the reference is to the end of the movement when energy is being expressed. Now, the striking part of the body may be more yang than another part of the body but overall the body's minimum yang-ness needs to be greater than that of the opponent.

To follow this point further, the hands during the movement associated with the application of the form are soft and rounded. Fair Lady's Wrist is maintained during the movement. At the moment of the strike, the body activates with the big toe on the rooted foot. The energy moves through the body to the hands, up to the fingers, and to the non-rooted foot. In this manner, the body is balanced and any part of the body can strike upon contact with the opponent. The player never thinks, "I am throwing a straight punch to the jaw" but extends and waits for the contact in the hollows of the opponent's attack and strikes upon contact. Many times Grandmaster Chen will demonstrate this by hitting the body with a number of shots, only one will have energy in it. The energy cannot be seen, only the power of the dreaded impact after his completion of the series of punches. Softness until hardness is required. In addition, it is critical to remember that the Professor always said to neutralize with four ounces but to strike with the appropriate level of force.

When doing the form there are many instances when there are slight turns and twists of the hands that many people do not practice. It is essential to understand these and upon full understanding, the movements may become so negligible that they cannot be observed but they are still there internally. Grandmaster Chen and the classics talk of small turn - big spiral. This means to turn right to go left. We do every day but do not realize it. When reaching down for an object, notice the body turns and then when picking up the object the body turns the other direction. It has been investigated in modern exercise and is discussed as a pre-stretch action. What it accomplishes in gross movements is to stretch the muscle that is to be contracted before its use. Since muscle cells can only contract, a pre-stretch extends more muscle cells before the action. When the action takes place, more cells can then contract making the movement stronger.

Now in Tai Chi Chuan this is only a part of the movements. As an example the application of brush knee is done with the hands circling one hand up and one hand down then one hand down and one hand up to perform the application. The first movement cannot be thought only as a preparation movement. It has a large number of application including a roundhouse punch or a back fist or even a throw. The hand being alive and turning as the hands move through the circle is essential if energy needs to be expressed during the first part of the movement. Some of these movements will be shown later but it is essential to understand every small movement of the form and its practical application. Break the form down to each movement and practice that movement until all its options have been found and then start again. See the Tui Shou volume and Appercise section for more details.

No Hand Business

Grandmaster Liang would also say this. It is only when you realize that the hands are moved in conjunction with the body. No body movement no hand movement. This is so that the Ch'i can flow from the root out to the hand and fingers. Any movement by the hand or the foot does not contain power unless it is connected to the body. This extraneous movement is seen in the Wu Shu forms where flourishes are added to make the form look pretty. He was always about business. If it moved it needed to be for a reason and that reason usually hurt. So, every movement that is in the form or practice must be traced through the body and into the root.

Eye focus

When doing the form or playing, the eyes should be gazing to the far horizon. This allows the body to relax and the gaze will be soft. When playing in this manner the eyes will recognize movement much quicker since the peripheral vision picks up movement faster when the gaze is unfocused. The eyes are also a source of energy control in the body. The eyes are associated with the upper burner. The eyes can assist directing the energy to the location impact. The eyes must remain soft in their gaze not a stare.

Gaze like a hawk

This does not contradict the previous item. If you gaze like a hawk all through the form you risk damage to your system. You will not be relaxed and you not be able to let the Ch'i flow. If, however you gaze like a hawk when attacking the target you will be as accurate and powerful as a hawk! This is the focus part of the art. The eyes remain soft and unfocused while doing theform allowing the relaxation of the body and mind. When it is time to express energy, the body must be activated and that is through the mind and the point of ficus becomes through the eyes with a defined focus on the attack. This only occurs during the attack and then the focus relaxes. Otherwise the risk of tunnel vision can compromise the ability to respond. In Tai Ch'i Chuan, the eyes are only one part of the practice. The eyes provide feedback on what is happening around the player. The player must also use all other the other senses to react. The focus of the eyes aids in the direction of the energy that comes from the Yi – mind.

Burn up to flame not down to ash

Assuming and holding a posture is a good way to practice Tai Chi Chuan. Minor adjustments and relaxations are made until the body and stance come together to form the posture. One of the faults in this process is when concentrating on the sinking of the Ch'i, the player sinks lower and lower into the ground losing the energy in the posture. Since the ending of a movement is an energy action, the body should expand and fill with Ch'i. The image of fire is frequently used. Concentrate at the point of ignition where the flame reaches up. When the flame is out all that is left is the ash. Maintain the flame and let it flare. Think about this phrase, put it into practice, and feel that surge of Ch'i.

Turn to the left and spin to the right

A basic principal of movement is to turn one way and then turn back the opposite direction. This is referred to as the pre-stretch. This has multiple benefits. First is the action of releasing the muscle. That action is a pre-stretch. This allows the muscle cells to release and stretch. A muscle can only contract. It does this by contracting individual cells and shortening up its length. When the muscle is initially relaxed, more cells are stretched and this allows them to participate in the action of the muscle when contracting. All the relaxing practice in Tai Chi Chuan allows the muscles to relax and stretch. More muscle cells that are relaxed allow any action to be stronger by the participation of those additional cells in a contracting action.

In addition, a turn becomes a neutralization and then changes into a spinning attack. This allows the opponent to attack emptiness and find fullness upon the return. The body turns to the left neutralizing the attack. When the opponent retreats the spin going to the right, follows and attacks him.

Spin the board

Place a thin board on the floor. Step on it with the weighted foot. Play a posture with the foot on the board. The foot spins inward to the center line when the toes activate for the movement. The board should spin also. Practice this and check the alignment of the knee at the end of the movement. Always spin into the structure of the body. This brings the knee into alignment and prevents stress to the outside ligaments of the knee.

Trust yourself – single weighted

We live on two legs. Tai Ch'i Chuan requires the use of those two legs but also requires an understanding of the root concept. Tai Ch'i Chuan requires a continuous root. The root can be switched to either foot but needs to be a single root into the ground. Why? Tai Ch'i Chuan uses neutralization throughout the form. Yes, two legs are strong but they limit the movement of the body both in movement forward and back and in turning. This concept goes against the grain for many practitioners. The understanding is slowly developed when you begin to trust having one rooted foot and allow the other to add to the energy of that root or to enable a rapid change in position and repositioning of the root in the free leg. In the Tui Shou volume, applications and practices for this concept will be available. Try and trust yourself that you can root when needed on the single foot and see the added functionality to your form.

Ratchet

The turning of the waist can be compared to a racket wrench. The wrench turns one way clicking as it turns but without any resistance. Once turned, it turns back with all the force generated by the reverse turn. The waist does the same. This is also related to the preloading procedure. In the classics – turn one way to go another.

Bouncing a ball

Bounce a ball on the floor and see how it comes back up – higher and higher when more force is applied. This is a mental concept to think of the ball just before expressing energy. Do not let the legs raise. The compression will be lost. Just image the energy coming back up from the floor. When shifting the weight to the foot, think of breaking the floor.

Straight vs circle

Tai Chi is noted for its circles. Many of them become smaller as experience grows but the masters do not go back to a straight line. Why is the curve better? Not only from a martial aspect but also from the health benefits, a curve is going to provide the best benefits.

First, from a martial point of view, the curve gives an infinite number of varying vectors in the power stroke. Consider the straight punch. The fist comes straight out and impacts the body with the power vector running down the arm and into the target. When using the curve even on what looks to be the straight punch, the base of the vector remains constant but as the hand moves through the circle the vector is at varying degrees of angle until the hand reaches the target. The hand can at any moment of the circle encounter an opposing force or a moving target. That point becomes the end point of the power vector of the punch.

When using circular movements, the body can adjust and release power throughout the circular movement. With enough development the power can be converted into a folding technique and express power in the same manner into any target when following the circle when using a folding technique. The angle of attack allows for a full power. A straight punch in this instance is like the side of an arrow and the punch is deflected with a full disposition of the power into nothingness. Using a straight line punch can only follow that vector.

The health benefits of the circle are subtle but when the body is analyzed during the movement the benefits can be seen. A joint that is used in only a straight line continually moves in the same manner and range. Usually this is a range used in the same day to day efforts. When using a circular movement the joint uses a larger range of motion and allows the exertion to be divided on all surfaces within the joint. This means less wear on any part of the joint. Also, the movement over the range of the joint increases the movement of the synovial fluid[17] in the joint sac that provides nourishment and lubrication to the cartilage that covers the surface of the bone in the joint and prevents bone on bone movement. Bone to bone connections occurs when the cartilage is worn away due to injury or repetitive movement and that bone to bone connection leads to a deteriorated bone surface and arthritis.

Circular movements also allow for more flow of the fluids in the body due to the greater movement of the joint and less compression to nay point when using a circular movement.

Tennis ball in the arm pit

The armpit needs to open to let the shoulders assume their proper position. Use a tennis ball to practice this action. The ball goes in the armpit that has to open to make room for the ball. Hold the ball while practicing postures. The mind will develop the engram required to maintain this position in the form.

Lines and Channels

There is much confusion in how energy is moved and regulated through the body. Many people want to push their Ch'i through the acupuncture channels when they should be looking to move the Ch'i through the joints and sinews. What does this mean? Think of the acupuncture channels as the control system of the body. Each point that is needled is a switch that adjusts the flow just as if it was a switch in an electrical system - an adjustable switch so the flow is regulated.

The Ch'i that we express as a force upon the opponent in the martial aspects of Tai Chi Chuan moves on the outside of the bones and through the sinews and past the joints. This only works when the body is relaxed and the joints open. Just like a steam system that heats the house, the Ch'i is the steam and it moves out on the outside surface of the bones and through the joints in the sinews. Once the energy is expressed, it is like the steam giving off the heat in the radiator. The steam then condenses to water and moves back to the source. Well, some of the Ch'i on the outside of the bones seeps into the bone hardening the bone and then into the marrow. After many times of moving, the Ch'i in the marrow begins to harden and feel like steel. Many times Grandmaster Liang would talk about this whole process and what those few masters, who managed to complete the circle of Ch'I, felt like when they laid an arm on you. He stated that the Professor had reached this height of practice. When the Professor laid his arm on you it was soft on the outside but carried a great weight like it was steel inside and drove you to the floor. This was the correct flow of the Ch'i when using the idea of the Rice pot[18].

Therefore, even though the Acupuncture channels have Ch'i flowing through them and can be impacted by an input of Ch'i like that of a strike, you need to understand that there is a flow of the martial energy through the body also. There are also points not associated with acupuncture points that can be impacted by a strike but that is only for advanced students and private instructions. Remember, that the best practice is the whole Tai Chi Chuan system and the use of a qualified Traditional Chinese Medicine doctor to administer needles. The Acupuncturist will help you achieve a proper flow and allow for the adjustment of any issues that develop in practice. More on this in the second Tai Ch'i Chuan volume.

Fa jin – An jin

Energy is energy. The expression of that energy takes one of two forms in Tai Ch'i Chuan – fa or an. Fa Jin is an explosion. An Jin is a bulldozer. The method of discharge is the length of time to express the energy. The Yang form practices the form with An as the normal energy action. The movement of a push visualizes the movement of an object with the intent of a change in position. The Fa energy can be practiced outside of the form. Fa expresses either as an imaginary action or upon a specific target as in strikes against a sand bag. Too much Fa practice is detrimental. So practice with this understanding. More on this issue is discussed in the other Tai Chi Chuan volumes and yes there are more types of energy. That is for the next volume.

Stance and Posture

The only way to get the information on these two parts is to describe the final picture and then talk about getting there. The stance is the lower body consisting of the feet and legs up to the kua – the kua being the joint of the hip. The pelvic girdle, the spine, the shoulders and the arms complete the stance. The posture is the position and purpose that the weapons of the body used while attached to the stance. The whole process of getting into the stance and assuming the posture is the movement.

Developing a root

Just as a tree has roots, the Tai Chi player must develop a root. The concept is the same as for a tree. The tree's root proves nourishment and connection to the ground. The Tai Chi Player's root provides nourishment of the Chi and stability of the body. Just as a deeply rooted tree does not topple, the Tai Chi Player should have a deep root and not topple either.

Rooting is a complex process but the heart of the process is simple – the relaxation into the earth. Most of the effort in generating a root comes from the control of the mind. When the mind is calm and relaxed yet bright and aware, the player can visualize the root and feel the earth. Once the mind is in the proper state, the player then practices techniques to allow the body to hold the root and prevent anyone from moving the player.

When discussing the root here, the focus is on single weighted stance vs a double weighted stance. The Professor has stated that the root is a single weighted stance. The root is with one foot. As Grandmaster Chen said, you must "trust yourself" to use only one leg to support the body. There are many benefits of this posture including better balance, less chance of falling, and from the martial side easier neutralization.

The various stances are defined and discussed elsewhere. The root starts with the foot. The foot needs to be flexible and able to open and close the joints within the foot. When the weight is on the outside of the foot the foot is not stable and rooted. Once the weight is transferred to the inside of the foot, the bones and joints of the foot lock and provide a solid foundation into the earth which gives the player the ability to establish a strong root. The knee turns inward slightly providing more stability to that joint.

When the root is established, the body position always maintains a center over the weighted foot. The body is light and flexible but as it bends as in a willow, the weight is still maintained over the foot by the movement of the hips, knees, and ankle.

This allows the player to bend far backwards in avoiding a push or punch but to maintain stability with movement of the hips. Also, be aware that the foot maintains a support posture but is also movable with the weight shifting between the three nails and the ankle becomes more flexible as the root grows in strength. See the exercises below for practice methods.

Stepping

The feet are adjusted to have the toes pointing forward when in the horse stance. The distance the feet are apart in an internal style is easy to determine with a broomstick handle. Put the base at the inside arch of the foot and the stick should pass through the nipple. Next, the bow stance needs to be practiced. Again, the front toe is pointing straight to the front with the rear foot being pointed out away from the body at an angle between 30 and 45 degrees. Yes, old style Yang form had the foot out at a 90-degree angle at times. There are places in the form where this is still done. A lessor angle allows for a freer movement of the energy and a proper positioning of the knee. The foot connects to the body and the knee moves inward. Actually, concentrate on the knee coming in by way of the hip moving forward and let the foot follow. **The hip is moving the foot -** When stepping the initiation of a step is through the movement started in the hip. The hip maintains the connection to the pelvic girdle. The alternate hip is the pivot point of the movement with the action hip lifting the leg from the floor and moving it forward. This keeps the whole body as part of the step and not a foot leading the parade.

Pivoting

The foot pivots throughout the form to assume the correct position in relation to the body. The foot pivots either on the toe or on the heel. A simple release of the toe or the heel will allow the pivoting of the foot. Seldom is the foot picked up off the ground and moved. The body should move the foot whether it is a pivot or placement. The form volume[19] will discuss each of these movements. The player should practice the turning of the foot both on the toe and on the heel. Many times the foot is picked up but that allows a possible sweep and should be considered in the application of the movement. Does it need to be up off the ground or can the foot maintain contact? When practicing the unweighted foot find that the toe gains upward energy and the heel gains downward energy. Think of this as you practice and more of this in the Tui Shou Volume.

Step lightly

When stepping forward or back, the foot is placed lightly on the ground – heel to toe when going forward and toe to heel when stepping back. This allows the player to feel the ground before placing any weight on the foot preventing a heavy weighted step upon insecure ground resulting in a fall. Also with martial implications, a foot sweep is more effective on a weighted foot. Stepping with weight allows the other player to time the step and sweep before a root is obtained.

Heel to toe - Stepping forward the heel should touch down first, assess the footing, and then roll into the rest of the foot. Roll to the outside and then shift to the inside of the foot. This is using the third nail that is the rooting portion of the foot and is considered home. Then moving into the front of the foot for action activities.

Outside to inside – The foot needs to go heel to toe. This type of step allows the foot to gain a grip on the ground. As the foot rolls out towards the toe, the weight is slowly applied to the outside of the foot. The weight opens the joints of the foot spreading the sole out and pushing down like a suction cup. When the weight is fully applied, the close contact of the relaxed foot allows the three nails to grip the ground and provide a powerful root. Upon initiation of an action, the weight shifts to the inside of the foot and knee rotates inward. When the weight is on the inside of the foot it locks all the joints of the foot into a single strong point and allows the power of the root to travel up the leg.

Foot slightly inward for a brake

The feet are parallel in the beginning of the form and any movement that involves the horse stance. In the bow stance, the forward foot is pointing forward and the rear foot is at an angle – in the Grandmaster Chen form, it is a 15 to 30-degree angle. Tai Chi Chuan as a martial art alters the forward foot slightly inward. This serves as a brake on the movements involving a waist turn and prevents the knee from turning outward and potentially stressing the ligament. This also provides more power in a punch or push. This is elaborated in the volume on Tui Shou and San Shou.

Knees go inward

The knees should on any action move inward – toward the body's center. This brings the knee above the inside arch of the foot. This stabilizes the knee centering it directly in line with the lower leg bones. The energy comes up through the foot into a stabilized knee and passes into the thigh. Moving the knee inward helps the foot shift the weight to the inside arch and that locks all the joints of the foot together to provide a strong root and allow the flow of energy through the foot.

The forward Stance

The forward stance has two positions – the ready position and the action position.

Ready Position

The ready position consists of a forward weighted position. The weight is on the front foot with only the weight of the rear leg remaining on the back foot. This is frequently referred to as 80/20 position. The weight should be on the outside edge of the foot. The three nails are attached to the floor but the heel nail is very lightly attached. The front foot should be toed in slightly no more than 30-degree angle. The leg is relaxed with the thigh held just over the center of the foot at a 30-degree angle from the horizontal with the knee over the big toe. The hip joint is relaxed allowing the upper body to tilt forward – the nose no further than the knee. The rear leg is up to a line directly under the body thigh straight down with the foot relaxed and the toe touching the floor. The heel may be off the floor but no effort should be in raising it. The knee of the rear leg should be just behind the front knee and the thigh in a straight downward position to the floor. The pelvic girdle is open and relaxed sinking down into the hip joint. The spine is tilted neither right or left and slightly bent and loose. The shoulders are dropped allowing the ribs to rise upward.

If the shoulders are raised the scapula will form an angle directing the energy and weight into the spine. This will put pressure on the base of the neck and the upper back and prevent the spine from raising upwards. The kua of the arm – the arm pit- is open which allows the shoulders to open up and away from the body. When this occurs, the scapula pulls away from the spine and allows the spine to remain loose and movable. The head sits squarely on the spine tilted neither right nor left with the chin tucked in slightly which helps to raise the occipital. Practice all of this!

Action Position

Tai Chi Chuan does not require a lot of movement to complete its action. The components connect to provide the force required from the root. This is accomplished in the following sequence. The big toe (little brain) activates by a turning inward and digging into the floor. The weight shifts on the front foot from the outside of the foot to the inside of the foot. This allows all the joints of the foot to lock into one solid brace to the floor. The bubbling well takes the energy from the root up through the body each of the joints remaining flexible to allow the energy to flow up. The legs are energized and filled with energy but do not extend upward. The energy is transferred through the kua to the upper body with the kua opening and the upper body straightening up as it fills with energy. The energy flows into the body filling it in all parts. The part that is attacking – in this case say the hand, receives the energy coming down the arm through the wrist – held in fair lady's posture and fills the fingers of the hand. The energy has also filled up the other hand and rest of the body but only through the use of the mind's intent. The activated hand expresses the energy out and into the target.

Rear weighted stances
Ready Position

A rear-weighted stance uses the same principles as the forward stance. There is the 80/20 weight distribution with the weight on the back foot. The toe, knee, and nose alignment are the same but for the back foot while the front foot remains in the front. The only real difference is that there are limited movements backwards so the front foot must be ready to assist. The front foot can assume either a toe down or heel down position on the floor. This provides stability without commitment. At any time, the foot can be moved to another location and a weight shift used to neutralize or attack. The front foot whether using a toe or heel position should have the sole just slightly off the floor to remain in a relaxed state.

Action Position

Back weighted positions are usually defensive or transitional to attack posture. For the defensive position the movement is limited so either the energy directed in by an attack is rooted into the rear foot or the body turns on the root of the rear foot. This is seen in the roll back posture where there is a need for the root but the posture deflects the attack into a void[20]. The rear foot moves into the rooted foot's inside edge to get the full rooting capability and the third nail (home)[21] is used to take any residual energy into the root. We see the offensive capability in repulse the monkey where the strike comes out from the read foot into the opposite arm. This is one area where cross the great river needs to be considered. The same arm and foot can be used but only with care since the action is on the same side and subject to a pull. More on this in the Tui Shou volume.

Posture

A posture is simply assuming the position with the body's weapons. This can be a single whip using a hook hand and a palm or a brush knee with two palms. The actions can be anticipated or completed. The energy comes out of the root through the stance and supplies the weapons with their energy. Just as a tank gets to the battlefield with a motor, transmission and body, the cannon then fires the projectiles that were carried there by the rest of the tank.

Single verses double weighted

You have two feet on the ground. If you put your weight, equally on both feet you are double weighted. If you put your weight on one foot you are single weighted. It is not as simple as that. The body is never just single or double weighted all of the time. It goes through phases where it is either one or the other in some divided percentage. It is important in how long the body stays either single or double weighted and how long and how to go from one posture to another.

When you are double weighed such as the first movement of the form, you have a strong and stable position. This is a position used frequently in exercise postures and standing meditation. It does have its defects though. It is a clumsy posture in that movement from it requires the shift of weight from the double weighted posture to a single weighted posture before any movement can be performed. There are also lines in which force directed at the player cannot be absorbed and the player is knocked over.

A single weighted posture is the weight all in one foot and the other foot has only the weight of the leg. This provides a strong weighted foot that gives a good root. The non-weighted leg can be moved without any weight shift so movement can be done as a change in leg position and a shift of weight. This allows for an easier neutralization of any force from any direction with either a turn of the body or a re-position of the un-weighted leg and a weight shift to that leg to avoid the force.

Trust yourself from the previous discussion. This was Grandmaster Chen way of getting the player to single weight and feel comfortable in a single weighted stance. Double weighted may feel stable and strong but it is clumsy and the player can easily be toppled. A single weighted posture is maintained in the Grandmaster Chen system. The single weighted system provides enough power to enable the posture in Tai Chi Chuan while maintaining a sense of mobility needed to neutralize as well as attack an opponent. A double weighted attack can be stronger but it is a clumsy force, not as well wielded, and subject to counter.

From a single weighted forward posture, the leg is pre-loaded. In effect, the gun is loaded, cocked, and ready to fire. To get to this position the weight is on the rear leg. The player steps forward heel to toe and shifts the weight into the forward leg that goes to a 90-degree angle at the knee – the knee not passing the toe. With the weight transfer, the player turns the waist to the side and bends a straight back down to a position to the bend position. The elbows open out to the sides and the hands stay close to the chest in a loose position.

The posture takes the concentrated power when the body is erected. The player releases the energy by erecting the spine and turning the body to face the opponent. The arms hold the energy and apply it to the opponent. The arms remain in the current position to hold the energy transferring it from the body to the opponent. If the arms move the compression of the energy will be released and not all directed into the opponent. Testing the technique is done using a chopstick. The arm should hold the chopstick in position unaffected by the force of the body and not dropped by the expanding arms. In practice once the energy is transferred through the arms into the opponent the arms stay in contact with the opponent to determine impact and any need for further action.

The Tui Shou section will discuss in detail the use of empty and weighted and the process of transition as it relates to practical use.

Stance Height

Many Tai Chi demo stances and forms have high stepping movements. This can make the form look very graceful and elegant. In Tai Chi Chuan, stepping needs to be considered in the martial aspect of the art. Keeping the foot close to the floor protects the root and prevents attacks to the raised foot that could topple the player. Sweeps, which are hidden in most of the movements, are able to attack both a weighted and a floating foot. If the body is rooted but not maintained in a posture centered over the root, an attacker can use that imbalance to move the body and sweep the foot. Moving with a high foot due to a high step can allow the opponent to use their foot or hand to get under the foot and due to the higher center of gravity with a raised leg, tip the player over.

The high stance is very effective in both Tui Shou and San Shou. When the feet are close, there is little time involved in changing the weight from foot to foot with limited body motion. Not only does this not telegraph the change in the rooted foot but allows for a rapid change back and forth. The shoeshine comes from the old boxers who took the example from the shoe shiners found on the corners in cities. The shoe shiners would take a shining rag and hold an end in each hand and buff with a cross body movement. Boxers, notably Sugar Ray, developed the technique and used it as a body attack coming from both sides. The art is to make each punch come from the rooted foot and the rooted foot changing back and forth with each punch. This makes a rapid attack of power punches that are fast and hard to defend. This technique is an example of why there is a close stance in the fighting style of Tai Chi Chuan.

The technique to use a short stance is to have the heel of the front foot only an inch or two ahead of the rear foot. The stance is not narrow with the normal foot position being just outside of the front channels but within the shoulder width. The forward/back position of the feet are closer. This provides a moving root. This is something that is not often used in Tai Chi Chuan. Many styles use an immobile root and attempt to neutralize around the root. This does work but many times requires the player to root all the force when the attack is not completely neutralized. Using a movable root provides more flexibility in movement. When a strong attack occurs the root as well as the body can be moved to avoid the attack. More on these techniques in other sections and the Tui Shou and San Shou volumes.

The Bows

The body is made up of a number of bows. Think of the analogy of a bow and arrow. From the joints of the hand to the whole body, the bow shape can be found. Test the power of the body expressed through the bows. A bow does two things - the first is to accept force into the body and dissipates that force into an arc. This allows the spring action to express the energy away from the body's center and prevent the energy from affecting the internal organs.

The second is an action of expressing force out using the power of the bend to act like a bow releasing the arrow. Sometimes this is the pre load of the player but many times is the stored energy from an attack directed back to the opponent. More on this subject in the other volumes.

Raise the head as if strung from a string

When raising the head most people stick the chin out. This tilts the head back. The thought must be to raise the head from the back and tuck the chin in. This action protects the chin but most importantly it opens the neck and the associated muscles and vertebrae. This is an essential area to keep the energy movement flowing.[22] The neck is also less likely to suffer injury. Being open and balanced, there is movement in all directions without immediately reaching a position where the movement is limited and injury to that area most likely.

Spine

The classics tell us that we must have a straight spine but like yin and yang, this is only one aspect of the spine in Tai Chi Chuan. When applying power; we must have a straight spine. This not only is a requirement from a physical point of view but also has impacts with Qi development and health.

If the spine is bent or misaligned when power is applied through it, the torque can cause the vertebrae to be deflected from their proper position and when this happens, the nerves can be pinched or a disc can be ruptured. None of this is good since most often this leads to a lifelong impact on the player's health. Also in the basics of physics, when the line of force does not follow a straight line - the spine – the multiple vectors of that force reduce the impact. This takes the power out of the application and most likely puts it into the player's body.

91

When the spine is in a straight line,[23] the power of the muscles flows up through the body. Muscles work on a simple contraction that prevents any torque in the muscles and provides the force in a direct line. All of these actions provides for a powerful movement.

When we talk about the movement of energy in the body, we also want to have a straight spine to keep the flow of energy from being impinged by any pinching of the energy channels. The action of a movement requires a large amount of coordination in the body. The first is the nervous system getting the command for action to the initial muscles. The supporting infrastructure such as the blood flow and the breathing is activated. This needs a tuned and flowing nervous system. The blood supply must also be reactive to a movement. Muscles require oxygen and glucose from the blood to make a movement. This has to be provided by the blood flow and then the waste products have to be removed immediately. Lactose, a byproduct of the muscle movement, is toxic and must be removed to prevent muscle exhaustion and cramping. At the same time, the lungs have to be moving the oxygen into the blood and removing the toxic gases. The liver and the kidneys must remove the wastes. Of course, there is time for an action to take place and all of these processes to complete. The body is made to have reserves and can survive without immediate removal of wastes. It is part of the art of Tai Chi Chuan to work with these systems on a daily basis. Bring these systems to the highest level of performance with the least amount of effort in either the practice of Tai Chi Chuan or the application of force.

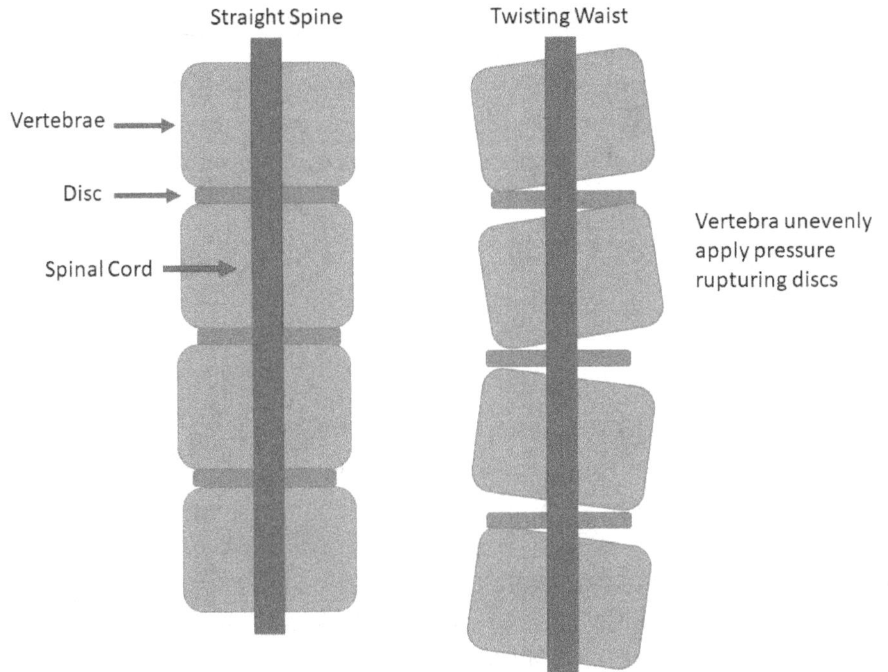

The time between the applications of force in the movements allows the spine to flex. This too can be used for martial purposes and for movement of the Ch'i. When someone pushes on the shoulder, shift all the weight back, and then turn the waist to neutralize the energy keeping the spine straight and follow the letter of the law in the classics.[24] The spine also is flexible and upon contact allows the shoulder to shift backward sectioning off the attached vertebrae in a turning movement that neutralizes the energy but keeps the player nearer to the opponent. The posture allows the player to have breached the defense of the opponent and then apply an attack to their center with the energy of the shoulder coming back into the spine and the spine now at a straight position directing the impact of the strike. This is the softness of Tai Chi Chuan turning into its hardness. Yin and yang in a balanced action.

Qi is energy and Qi requires channels[25] to flow through the body. The spine is one of these major freeways. The Qi flows through all the major channels using the spine – blood, lymph, nerves and one major one – the Cerebral Spinal fluid – the fluid in the spine that flows up and around the brain. This flow is extremely important to maintain the health of the central nervous system. The Cerebral Spinal fluid is replaced three times a day and provides not only a fluid channel for the waste products of the brain and the spinal cord but provides a cushioning effect on these systems. Since there is no particular organ that is responsible for the flow of this fluid, it uses various techniques to circulate and remove the fluid from the system. Just as lymph fluid moves about the body due to changes in body posture and muscle movement, the Cerebral Spinal fluid uses these and the lymph and blood systems to move in the body.

There is also the Cerebral Spinal pump[26] that can be developed to increase the flow in this system. When the body moves, the spine has movement also. This movement helps move the spinal fluid up to the brain. Every time we breathe in and stretch our spine, the spine elongates and upon relaxation, the compression of the spine pumps the fluid up to the brain. This process can be enhanced through the movements of Tai Chi Chuan. The relaxing and the straightening of the spine provides this same action and increases the flow of the Cerebral Spinal fluid. We can take this farther by doing exercises that stretch the spine (open) and relax the spine (close). When doing these actions, the vertebrae act as individual pumps and all contribute to the flow. The stretching of the spine increases the spacing of the vertebrae with the spinal disk expanding as the spine opens. Upon relaxation, the spine closes and the vertebrae come together decreasing the space in the spinal column and pushing the Cerebral Spinal fluid up the spine.

Shoulders

The shoulders must be relaxed but not slouching. There has to be enough energy in the shoulders to maintain their openings away from the spine. The gap, as discussed elsewhere, remains throughout the form. The shoulders are also square with the body creating the four corners. Attention is directed to the minor muscles that allow for the minor movements. These muscles relax allowing the movement of the shoulder in any direction. If the minor muscles are not relaxed, the movement of the shoulder is against a tightened muscle and may injure that muscle. These muscles do not heal rapidly and may retain injury related issues.

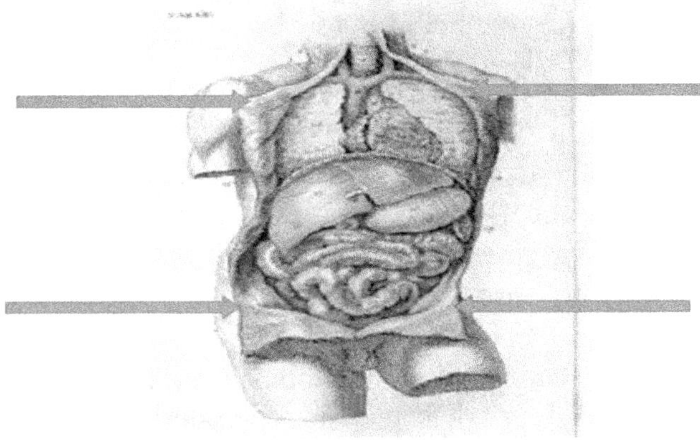

Shoulders are strengthened by continuous movements. Daoyin and Qigong as well as Ligong exercises provide fine conditioning options above and beyond the form.

Thorax

The thorax is the major structure of the body. Through it the energy from the legs and arms work. The thorax must be strong but relaxed. Straightness leads to a straight spine. The ribs protect all the organs of the body. Movement in the ribs is possible with relaxation. This prevents adhesion in the sinews. The flexibility of the thorax and within it the ribs, provides the ability to absorb impact force while protecting the organs. When the ribs relax, the inner gap between bones opens. This is most notable in the spinal connection. The spinal nerves that branch from the spinal cord have free flow when the ribs open and allow the vertebrae to open the space between them. The ribs are divided into two groups – fixed and floating. The fixed ribs are attached to bone front and back but have some movement with relaxed muscles and breathing. More importantly, the floating ribs can move down and away from the fixed ribs with body and muscle positioning providing for room and movement within the torso. [27]

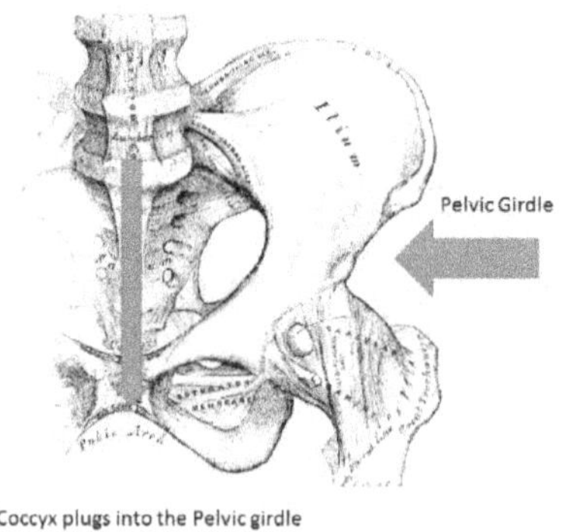

Coccyx plugs into the Pelvic girdle

Pelvic Girdle

Whenever talking about structure in Tai Chi Chuan, the critical component is the pelvic girdle. This is an apparatus of the body consisting of muscles, bones, ligaments, and tendons. They form the connection of upper and lower to complete the body structure. The pelvic girdle provides the connections between the thorax and the legs. The girdle is a moving connection that controls and connects the flow of not only the fluids of the body but the physical force and the Ch'i. The girdle can be thought of as two wings each composed of the coxal bones, a bone made of the fused bones ilium, ischium, and pubis that happens with maturity. Each of these bones can act as if on a hinge either together or independently. When moving in and out, they create a pump that creates pressure in the body and assists in the movement of the blood and lymph through the body. When playing Tai Chi Chuan, the movement of the hips becomes an essential component of the movements. When the stance is created, the hipbones allow the spine to plug into the pelvic girdle and create a connection between the power source of the root below and the expression above. The expression of energy in a movement such as brush knee and push is an example. The hip open as the body turns away and the hands turn over. As the brush and push come forward, the front hip pivots and draws the rear hip into the closure of the pelvic girdle. This increases the pressure in the body allowing the energy to be expressed out to the hands.

Legs

The legs are one of the strongest muscle systems in the body. We use them extensively. Tai Ch'i Chuan uses the strength of the legs to direct its force also but in another manner – stored energy. The legs can store a large volume of energy from their movements. This storage is like filing your tank with gas. You only use it when needed.

The legs initially are used to express energy out but with the development of a root and the ability to understand its use, the legs become the reserve and transport mechanism for the root energy. The legs are strong holding the energy as it is transferred from the legs into the upper body. The use of the natural bow created by the legs and their connection to the Kua make the whole body bow. The legs assume a posture with the natural bow and the connection through the foot to the root. The joints all remain relaxed and open. The toe initializes the energy exchange and the legs move slightly with the transfer of energy but must stay in their bow position to transmit that energy into the upper body. If the player raises up with the legs during an action, the energy will only be through the muscles of the legs and not the connection to the root. As the player works on the form and relaxation they will understand the difference and the increased level of power when the legs maintain a springy but shaped posture.

Feet

The principle of the three nails is unique to Grandmaster Chen system but is an essential concept in Tai Chi Chuan that Grandmaster Chen has been able to explain through this visual concept. The three nails - the big toe, the ball of the foot and the heel are all used to make the connection to the root energy and to express that energy into the body. The big toe, also called the little brain due to its influence in acupuncture, is used as a trigger or switch to initiate the energy flow. The valve opening to flow energy is the ball of the foot. In all instances of movement, the foot is turning inward. This is required to shift the weight to the inside of the foot and to allow the knees to move inward.

When the weight is on the outside of the foot, the foot relaxes and is soft and flexible. When the weight is transferred to the inside of the foot, the bones of the foot lock forming a single structure. This makes the foot structurally strong and allows the energy to be transferred to the body from the root. The knees moving inward make a stronger and less stressful stance. If the knees drift outward, the exterior ligament is subject to stretching and tearing. A ligament that is stretched does not come back to its original length. Too much stretching and the knee loses its support structure. Also with this energy movement, both knees are coming inward which focuses the energy up the legs and into the spine like pushing on the base of a loose pyramid and the top moving upward.

Back to the foot - the ball of the foot turning in and pushing downward allows the bubbling well to reach into the root and allows the transfer of energy into the foot.

Where is the third nail in this discussion? Think of it as home or a ground. After expressing energy, the body relaxes and the weight shifts backward located closer to the heel and the heel touches the ground. That allows the energy to flow back into the Earth. It is also used to reach the root when a force is applied and allows the foot to root and absorb that force preventing the player from being toppled over. When using the first two nails the heel actually may lose contact with the ground - slightly. From an electrically point think of making the opponent is the ground when expressing energy and all that energy goes into the opponent since the energy is coming up from the first two nails but there is no ground (third nail) so the opponent is electrocuted!

Toes

The toe is used to connect the foot to the ground and to trigger the connection from the body to the root through the foot. The big toe and depending upon the flexibility of the foot and the connection to the individual toes, the index toe, is activated, and presses downward and inward toward the center line of the body. This changes the weight from the outside of the foot to the inside and at that time the foot connects all the bones together into a stable and unmovable joint able to support the body weight and provide a connection to the root and floor.

This is where the power originates for the movement whether it is considered the physical connection to the floor or the energy connection through the bubbling well. The movement into the center of the body moves the knee slightly inward that stabilizes the knee and provides a strong base for the power triangle of the stance. This directs the energy to the apex of the pyramid where a movement to the outside would send the power away from the power pyramid.

Using the fingers and the toes as the brain of the body is a main fundamental technique of Grandmaster Chen. He has developed it to the point that the body follows the actions of the fingers with the toes applying the power when needed. This is a concept hard to understand for numerous martial artists that learn a fist as a strike. Once they clench the fist the biceps become active and slowing down the punch and restricting the power of the movement.

The Heel

Taking on the role of the third nail the heel is the home and safe spot grounding the body when required. When applying a movement, the heel gives up its attachment to allow the first two nails to express the energy in the movement. Yet when under attack the heel's nail is driven into the ground to provide a strong root. Many times in Tai Chi Chuan, we neutralize to avoid an attack. There are times when we cannot or do not want to neutralize. Then the heel nail attaches and provides a ground for that energy. We do use the other two nails to provide stability but the major energy flow is through the heel.

When making a large movement such as a 180 to a 360-degree turn, the heel is used due to its ability to retain a root while allowing the body to turn and spinning on the heel's nail. This is something that must be practiced to prevent injury. Many times movement of the foot on a surface can grab and cause a fall or even a knee injury. Allowing the front two nails to give up their connection and the third nail to spin can allow a turn on this type of surface without injury while still remaining in control. Try this on a carpet that does not let the foot adjust as the sole grabs. Spin by lifting the front of the foot and pivoting on the heel. The heel with practice can spin and allow a turn. Remember this also whenever a simple foot adjustment is needed. The security of the third nail can remain with the first two releasing allowing a change in foot position.

Fingers

The median and the ulnar nerves are the two main nerves that run through the fingers. Hold the upper arm in one hand and with the fingers of the other hand feel the connection to the upper arm muscle. When moving the thumb, index and middle finger feel the triceps activate. The movement will be slight so lightly hold the muscles. Using the ring and pinkie fingers, feel the biceps activate. The power movement of a muscle is to contract. Muscles have an opposite muscle that relaxes upon the contraction of the muscle. When using the thumb and two fingers, the triceps are activated and contract. This contraction directs the arm outward as the biceps relaxes and elongates. Using the last two fingers, the biceps contracts, and the triceps relaxes allowing the arm to move inward. Using this imagery, the player can see that the push – an away movement - is controlled by the fingers and thumb. A pull or grab such as used in a throw uses the last two fingers. Now there is more body mechanics involved in any movement but the control switch can be isolated down to the fingers and the toes (see below).

The thumb must be in alignment with the first and middle finger. This is the energy of the thumb directing the energy of the fingers. The fingers can curl as they strike the target but the energy will follow the direction indicated by the thumb.

The pinkie and the thumb can direct the energy flow and direction. This was explained above but try it again. Test this out. Squeeze together the thumb and first two fingers while having the other hand on the triceps. The muscle contracts. Do the same with the ring finger and the pinkie finger. The biceps contracts. A muscle can only apply force when contracting. So the direction of the first movement is outward and the second is backward. Think on this and see how it relates to you postures in the form. This is important. More on this in the other volumes.

Tai Chi Walking

Tai Chi Walking fits into the power walking mold. Most people will think that Tai Chi walking will be this slow motion walking but that is too limiting. Walking is one of the best exercises for the general population and should be practiced by everyone who can walk. With the knowledge of Tai Ch'i Chuan and its practices, the walking exercise can take on many flavors.

First is the speed. True walking should have many speeds and from research, interval training is best for development of the body. Well, walking has all the capabilities of interval training. But, first the basics

Walking should be done in a heel to toe step. The foot is raised with the rear foot peeling off of the ground from the heel lifting until the toe comes off the ground. The step length should be heel slightly in front of the toe of the opposite foot in a parallel position with the foot pointing straight ahead in the direction of the movement. The heel touches down and the weight is applied as the foot rolls into the toe. The actual weighting goes from the outside edge of the foot to the inside with the final weight in alignment with the ball of the foot.

The action of the foot in the peeling motion of both the rear step and the forward step is to flex the foot and allow stimulation of all the physical points in the foot. The foot is considered a main focus point in reflexology and acupuncture. Movement in the foot, which is usually bound up in too tight shoes with limited flexibility, will allow for the stimulation of these points. This will benefit the body during the walking. See also the information on the pump in the foot[28]. This movement is essential to get that action to its fullest potential.

While walking change he speed of the steps over intervals. Start slowly walking at the speed of Tai Ch'i Chuan and then speed up and slowly drop back down. This is repeated throughout the walk. Once straight line walking is easy, then add in cross step, and rear walking.[29] Rear walking works great with a partner. You can have a face to face discussion.

Stepping

Many Tai Chi demonstrations and forms have high stepping movements. This can make the form look very graceful and elegant. In Tai Chi Chuan, stepping needs to be considered in the martial aspect of the art. Grandmaster Liang always taught a close to the floor foot during any movements unless a raised foot was required within the movement such as a kick. Keeping the foot close to the floor protects the root and prevents attacks to the raised foot that would topple the player. Sweeps, which are hidden in most of the forms, are able to attack both a weighted and a floating foot.

If you have rooted but not maintained a posture centered over the root, an attacker can use that imbalance to move the body and sweep the foot. Moving with a high foot due to a high step can allow the opponent to use their foot or hand to get under the foot. Due to the higher center of gravity with a raised leg, the player is tipped over. Grandmaster Liang did this regularly to an opponent. Even keeping the toe raised at too high - a position off the floor in raise hands - and he would slide a foot under and tip you backwards. He stressed keeping the foot just off the floor to quickly regain a root, prevent exposure and most of all to maintain rooted and sunken Ch'i. Grandmaster Chen also has low foot positions mostly due to his closely placed foot positions in the form.

Grandmaster Liang kept what would be considered a middle stance in his form where Grandmaster Chen uses a high stance. This is very effective in both Tui Shou and San Shou. When the feet are close, there is little time involved in changing the weight from foot to foot with limited body motion. Not only does this not telegraph the change in the rooted foot but allows for a rapid change back and forth. See the Shoe Shine above

The technique is to use a short stance is to have the heel of the front foot only an inch or two ahead of the rear foot. The stance is not narrow with the normal foot position being just outside of the front channels but within the shoulder width. The position of the feet are close toe to heel. This provides a movable root. More on these techniques in other volumes.

Breathing

There are many techniques for breathing in the martial arts. In the Yang form, as taught by Grandmaster Chen, the breath is a major part of learning the form. He says everyone can breathe in since that is what a baby does at birth so he teaches the breathing technique that has a focus on controlled out breath. What does this mean? First we need to get some background on techniques.

Pre Natal and Post Natal Breathing

When the baby is in the womb, they are provided nourishment from the mother. This is provided from the connection of the umbilical cord. The gas exchange process – breathing – is taken care of by the mother. The baby's lungs are filled with the amniotic fluid. The baby learns to breathe while still in the womb but the breath is taken in with the pre-natal breathing method. This is where the abdominal section of the body is sucked in on the in breath. The baby when doing this draws blood in from the mother that has oxygenated blood and passes the waste gases off. Think of the umbilical cord as a straw. This form of breathing is used in some martial systems as well as in various Taoist yoga techniques.

The post-natal breathing technique is what we normally do to intake a breath. The chest and the abdominal cavity expand allowing the lungs to fill with air and make the gas exchange.

It would take a book to discuss the techniques for both of these systems and debate the pluses and minuses of each system. That will be in a subsequent volume. We will focus on what we use within this system which is the post natal breath used in an enhanced breathing process.

When doing the form, the breath is in just before the action and out on everything else. If you notice most of the time you take an in breathe quicker than you breathe out. Mostly this is due to the action of the muscles. The action of breathing[30] in requires an exertion of the muscles to create a vacuum that fills the lungs up with air. The lungs pass the air into the alveoli that transfer the Oxygen to the blood and absorb the waste gases from the blood. Breathing out in a sub conscious manner is just a relaxation of the muscles that allows the muscles to go back to their normal position expelling the air from the lungs. The blood gas exchange is a very complex process. It is is very interesting but beyond this document but we need to understand the process of getting the good air in and the bad air out.

The post-natal breathing process can be enhanced by the focus on the breath while doing the form. The concept is simple. The breath is out on all the relaxation movements and in on the preparation movements. If an action movement is applied the breath is held until the action is completed. The dynamics of the internal breathing process are in the next volume of this series.[31] Follow the below section for the basics.

Breathing Exercise

As Master Chen says we all know how to breathe in, we need to be taught to breathe out. From the first breath a baby takes to our everyday sighs we are breathing in. We now need to practice the breathing out incorporated into Tai Chi Chuan that allows the lungs to function in the exchange of gases. Breathing in is for one purpose – to provide oxygen to the body. With the lungs filling with air the oxygen is combined with the hemoglobin to be transported to the cells for the generation of energy. What also happens in this process is the release of gas byproducts during the air exchange.

Breathing is where we can make an improvement that helps the body function to its potential. The lungs are made up of a series of small balloon like chambers (alveoli) that are surrounded by capillaries filled with blood. As the air fills up these balloons, the oxygen is attached to the hemoglobin in the red blood cells and removed from the chamber. It is replaced by the waste gases which even out the pressure. Now as the air is exhaled the waste gases are incorporated in the unused air previously breathed in. This not only removes gases that are toxic to the body but also allows for the balancing of the body's PH or acid / alkaline balance.

Physically what happens when we breathe? The diaphragm, a flat band of muscle that separates the lungs from the other organs in the thorax (belly region) contracts pulling the muscle down from the lung region and creates a vacuum. Since the lungs in a healthy person are flexible, they expand into the vacuum. The outside air rushes in and fills up the space in the alveoli (balloons) with air. This is the intake of breathe. Use of other muscles can alter and enhance this process. More on that later. Once the breathe is in, the diaphragm relaxes and the air if pushed out by the combination of the muscle relaxing and the abdominal mass pushing back to its original position and the elastic nature of a balloon deflating due to pressures equalizing. This completes a normal breath cycle.

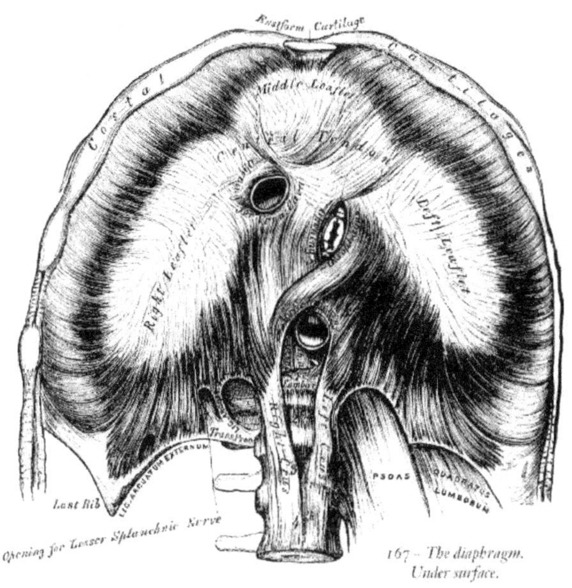

167 – The diaphragm.
Under surface.

One of the major problems with this process is that we rarely use the full capacity of the lungs. We take small intake and release breaths and this only uses the upper regions of the lungs. The alveoli in the lower lobes are there but infrequently used. They still have the ability to expand slightly with the increased pressure of the in breath and absorb waste gases into their cavities. Without the complete exhale, the gases stay in place and are not expelled. This creates an unhealthy area in the lungs that impacts the whole body. Not only are the lungs not removing the waste products to their greatest efficiency but also the habitat for growth of noxious organism is increased within the pockets of waste.

First the basic breathing process those players can take with them even if they leave the practice of Tai Chi. Later the detail how the breathing is used and impacts Tai Chi.

Either stand or sit depending on the health of the player. Take a series of deep breathes. No more than five or six. Remember this can impact blood pressure and cause a fall so keep it limited.

Next a series of sighs. Make note that the deep breath has a short exhale where the sign has a quick intake followed by a long exhale.

Next spend some time just watching and listening to the breathing. Once the mind focuses on the breathing, the autonomic nervous system gets trumped by the active brain.

Next ignore the in breathe and concentrate on the exhalation. Slow it down and feel the trickle of air going out. Not too much slowing down at first. Find the bottom of the breath cycle. After some time finding the normal bottom exhale slightly more when hitting the bottom. Where does this air come from? The unused alveoli are being squeezed to expel their toxic gases. If measured, the content of this last exhalation has a much higher level of waste gases. Note that after a few attempts the body will want to take in a large inhale. This is a normal reflex action from the brain and should be noted and encouraged as a part of the exercise.

Now with this background in place the exercise is very simple. Find a comfortable position and start concentrating on the breathing. Then transition to the focus on the exhalation. Slow it down and increase its length. When the body requires it take a large intake and breathe normally for a few cycles then go back to the trickle breath. This exercise should be practiced for 5- 10 minutes at most. Do not struggle or force the breath. Indicators for caution on this exercise are anyone with heart or blood pressure issues or anyone with asthma should only practice after a doctor's approval. Remember asthma is the inability to empty the lungs just what this exercise works on. The relaxation from this exercise can become therapy of the asthmatic spasm in the alveoli. This needs further research and doctor approval!

A variation after a few weeks of practice of the basic exercise is Grandmaster Chen's traveling breath. In the form there are points where he has an extremely long out breath that causes many people distress. He has changed this to what is the traveling breath. It is used when reaching the bottom of the exhale but there is more time before the inhale in the posture. A stoppage in the exhale and a relaxation of the body allows a slight in breath caused by the external air pressure. This generates the availability of external oxygen without a complete in breath. The player can travel through the form while this is happening or even start exhaling again. This provides for long out breathes which empty the lungs and can refresh the body as the clean air comes into the empty lungs with the next in breath.

Developing a root
Standing exercise

The standard standing exercise [32] is a very good method of developing the root along with its other benefits. As one stands the legs become stronger and can become more flexible. The visualization is of relaxing into the ground and developing an extended connection into the earth. Since standing exercise is not static, micro adjustments of the body will prepare it for the neutralization in push hands.

Neutralization Exercises

The neutralization exercises not only teach you how to neutralize an attack. They allow the practice in a relaxed manner, the movements that are required to maintain a root. As a partner pushes the player, relaxation and the partner's support allows for greater movements and the development of the body's ability to manage those movements.

Pushing exercises

When practicing pushes the B partner is usually called the dummy since they are taking the push without attempting to neutralize it. When practicing there should be a light body as well as a heavy body technique. When using the light body, the dummy still practices rooting but practices control of the root allowing the push and rooting after the push. With the heavy body – practice rooting with the push so your player gets to practice on a weighted body as well as uprooting techniques. The dummy gets to practice rooting and the varying degrees of root to use.

Root Transfer

The root of the player is critical to the practice of Tai Ch'i Chuan and where and how the root is used. The establishment and transfer of the root will be discussed here with the concept of the bow stance in a forward and backward position. The stance and transfer is the object of discussion and not the upper body that will be covered later. This section will describe the transfer as best as possible with words. The use and movement is only mastered with practice and following the rules until the player's body does the action without thought.

Assume a left footed back weighted posture. (left foot is in the front). A line on the floor either drawn or using lines of tiles can assist in managing the practice. The rear right foot is directly under the body and turned out from the center line 30 degrees. The left foot is facing directly forward flat on the floor with no weight on it. The distance between the feet is shoulder width apart and the heel of the front left foot is two to three inches ahead of the toes of the rear right foot.

The right rear foot is the rooted foot at this time. The foot is relaxed but the weight is on the inside edge of the right foot. This makes the joints of the foot stable and able to maintain the stance. The transfer of the root to the front foot begins with the big toe of the right foot. It is considered the "little brain" and activates by pushing down and scooping up the floor. Try in sand using the foot bare and scoop up sand with the foot acting like your hand. This is the action required to start the energy transfer from the floor to the stance. As the energy starts to activate in the right leg, it moves up the leg through the joints to the hip. Each joint opens slightly with the flow of energy. At no time does the leg erect itself. It just becomes filled with energy and pressure builds up in the leg. This allows the hip joint to begin moving weight from the weighted right side towards the left side. This energy flows through the pelvic girdle and into the left hip and then down the leg. The left foot begins to take on the pressure of the body going into the outside of the foot. The knee is important at this time. It must stay in line with the center of the foot. Do not allow it wander outward since this will put strain on the ligaments of the knee.

When the weight is transferred over to the left foot, the foot shifts the weight to the inside edge of the foot. This locks the foot in and allows for the connection to the floor and the root. Energy just enough to hold the posture in place is extended up the left leg. While the shift of weight is moving out of the right side to the left foot, it loses its root to the floor and becomes unweighted. The left knee moves forward to the center of the left foot. The right knee moves closer to the left weighted and rooted knee until the right thigh is straight down.

This is a simple movement but must be practiced until perfected. While in the transfer process, the player is susceptible to being pushed since there is a moving root. As a player, this is a time when your opponent is at their weakest and you should be aware of any changes such as this. Practice it slowly in the form and while playing in a two person set. Once the process is understood then the speed can be increased and a root transfer can be instantaneous.

When transferring to the unweighted foot, that foot must be relaxed to receive the energy. The foot is only relaxed when on the outside edge since the joints can be opened. If the foot is not relaxed, the energy will bounce back and aid in the opponent toppling the player over as the energy does not root but comes back up. Think of the Pogo stick or an inflated ball. They bounce! You will too if you don't receive the energy properly. Even the leg must be relaxed and the joints open and relaxed for the energy to flow through them. After the root is obtained the leg then become supportive and capable of expressing energy. If this transfer of root is not practiced slowly and properly then the player will never be able to transfer the root instantaneously as required in true playing.

Transferring the root from a front leg to the rear leg follows the same process but with the forward knee moving backwards and the back knee moving over the center of the foot. The back foot then attaches to the root by shifting to the inside edge of the foot.

Maintaining a root consists of the weighted foot maintaining the inside edge of the foot being connected to the floor and enough energy from the floor (root) to maintain the stance on the rooted leg. Only when energy is needed is there a activation of the toe drawing energy up from the root. This can be for a change in the root or for a posture action.

Remember:

- Tony Knows (Toe Knee Nose)

- Perpendicular thigh

- Big toe activate the process

- Shift outside of foot to inside to grab a root

- Relax everything remember softness

Do not:

- Scoop with little toe – the weight will go to the outside edge of the foot and the knee will move outward. The body will lose its center and fall to that side with little effort of the opponent.

- Allow the knee to wander out from the foot.

Horse Stance

The horse stance is the standard stance that runs through all the martial arts. Tai Ch'i Chuan uses it in a different manner than most in that it is a single weighted stance to conform to the idea of a single weighted root. Horse stance is only 50\50 at the beginning of the form before the differentiation of the yin and Yang. Afterwards it is only 50\50 in the middle of a transition movement and at that time it presents a weakness in the stance. The weight will always be 80\20 at any holding of the stance. This provides differentiation of the yin and yang energy.

The transition for one leg to the other in the horse stance is performed in the same manner as in the bow stance but the direction of transition is laterally across the body. The stance is with both feet at shoulder width apart and the toes directly forward. The weight on the left foot – in this example – is on the inside edge of the left foot. The toes and the arch of the foot hold the main portion of the weight. The heel is lightly attached and is not holding any substantial amount of weight. The right foot is flat on the ground with only the weight of the leg but it too only has weight on the front 2/3 of the foot with the help of the ground. The left foot then begins the transition with the big toe scooping and pressing down to get the energy of the root into the left leg and up into the waist. The weight transfers through the pelvic girdle into the right hip and down the leg into the right foot. The right foot takes the weight to the outside edge of the foot. This allows the foot to remain relaxed and absorb without the weight bouncing back. Once the weight is transferred the right foot shifts into the inside edge and connects to the root on the right side. The left foot remains in the same location but the weight is no longer in the leg. This transition must be practiced until the change in the root can not be seen externally. As it is practiced the speed in which the root can change is increased until it is instantaneous.

The stance is used to start the form and end it in a double weighted manner and can be used in this manner for developing the body. Part of the initial training in the original Tai Ch'i Chuan required many hours of training in the horse stance. Below is an exercise from those early texts that is quite valuable to make part of your regular training exercises. This exercise is also included in the Golden Flower Daoyin volume

- Posture and attitude

- Feet pointing to the front parallel just shoulder width apart

- Weight is 50 / 50

- Knees slightly bent

- Upper body is upright with a slight relaxation at the kua

- The head is up and the eyes looking forward chin not protruding

- Relax the chest and drop the shoulders

- The back is straight with its normal bends

- Elbows slightly dropped

- Tailbone is tucked in taking some of the arch out of the lower back

- Breath through the nose.

- Both arms are out in front of the body at shoulder height rounded like wrapped around a ball palms inward.

Take an in breath

Release the breath as the knees bend and you squat down keeping the back straightened

Maintain your center by shifting the weight forward by bending at the kua

Sit as if you were sitting into a chair.

Stop at the level of a chair with the thighs parallel to the ground.

Do not let the knees either go past the toes or to wander from directly above the footprints

As you go down your arm circle relaxes and grows slightly smaller and the elbows sink downward

Hold at the end of the breath for a second or two.

Gradually breathe back in raising yourself with the energy of the breath to the starting position.

The arms fill up and out with the imaginary ball growing fuller with the in breathed

Stop at the top let the breath have time to fill the body and then resume the out breath as you repeat the cycle.

After practicing for a while and the legs growing stronger imagine the energy coming up the spine with the in breath and sinking down the front of the body to the Tan Tien (elixir field) [33]

Other thoughts on Rooting

Using a tackling sled or other heavy movable object can develop your strength for a push and with your focus on your root. Know that you will just get strength in your push if you do not focus on the root as you use your strength.

Just as a tree has roots the Tai Chi player must develop a root. The concept is the same as for a tree. The tree's root proves nourishment and connection to the ground. The Tai Chi Player's root provides nourishment of the Chi and stability of the body. Just as a deeply rooted tree does not topple the Tai Chi Player should have a deep root and not topple either.

Rooting is a complex process but the heart of the process is simple – the relaxation into the earth. Most of the effort in generating a root comes from the control of the mind. When the mind is calm and relaxed yet bright and aware the player can visualize the root and feel the earth. Once the mind is in the proper state the player then practices techniques to allow the body to hold the root and prevent anyone from moving the player.

When discussing the root here the focus is on single weighted stance vs a double weighted stance. The stances are defined and discussed elsewhere. The root starts with the foot. The foot needs to be flexible and able to open and close the joints in the foot. When the weight is on the outside of the foot the foot is not stable and rooted. Once the weight is transferred to the inside of the foot the bones and joints of the foot lock and provide a solid foundation into the earth that gives the player the ability to establish a root.

When the root is established the body position always maintains a center over the weighted foot. The body is light and flexible but as it bends as in a willow the weight is maintained over the foot by the movement of the hips knees and ankle.

This allows the player to bend far backwards in avoiding a push or punch but to maintain stability with movement of the three joints. This also allows for a quick response since there is no need to shift the weight before initiating an action.

Explanation of the Basic Postures

An explanation of the basic stances and postures – movements[34] - found throughout the various Tai Chi hand forms are described in the following section. The focus of the method of playing the form is from Grandmaster Chen's system. This will provide the player with guidance in the principles of each movement and allow for corrections of the form. The postures will be discussed individually rather than as a string of postures in a form. Added to these descriptions are some postures that are seen in other Yang Tai Chi Chuan styles but have not been used in Grandmaster Chen's form. There are a number of other postures that are not part of this discussion on the form. They appear in the Da Lu and Tai Chi Chuan Dance sets and are discussed in those volumes. The advanced volume of the Golden Flower Tai Chi Chuan Series[35] will present the martial use of postures, the energy movements in the body and the intricate movements so that the player can advance in the practice of Tai Chi Chuan. These descriptions are for basic understanding of the posture. Detailed instructions are in volume three of this series and application are in Tui Shou and San Shou volumes.

Excellent descriptions and pictures are available in Grandmaster Chen's book - Body Mechanics of Tai Chi Chuan

Evaluating Your Postures

Tai Chi Chuan requires the evaluation of the body and mind at all times. The postures are played in the form, in combined sets and alone for this evaluation. The important points will be discussed here. They are only the basics and with practice, more corrections are always waiting.

Stepping

The foot always steps to the heel in a forward direction and to the toe on a rearward step. The foot is kept soft and flexible during a step. The weight shifts into the foot weighting the outside edge first and then shifting the weight to the inside arch to express energy. The three nails discussion explains the use of the nails during the stepping process.

Knees

The knees must stay over the foot and above or slightly forward of the toes on a weighted position. The alignment of the knee is always over the foot until the expression of energy. At that time, the knee moves slightly inward to protect the ligaments from damage.

Breathing

Breathing is always soft and controlled. The out breath is used throughout the movement and an in breathe allows for the collection of energy. Hold the breath upon application of energy.

Softness

Always look for more softness in the body when assuming a posture. Only enough muscular energy is used to maintain the posture. Stop when working on a posture and evaluate all the muscles holding the body. Especially look at the pelvic girdle for more muscles that can relax.

Posture

The posture during a movement is relaxed and flexible. There is no straightness in the body. There are also no disjointed movements. Upon assuming the posture, the body straightens. The head and spine are upright and in alignment. The torso is plugged into the pelvic girdle and the legs are in supporting positions.

Timing

Movement from one posture to the next starts with the fingers. The fingers release the body and move everything to the position where the next step may be taken. The body moves into the base of the posture and the toes take over, initiate the movement, and connect back to the fingers. Everything between the fingers and toes just follow their direction.

Holding the Ball is the mother – Ward Off is the Father

Holding the ball is seen in transitions throughout the form. It is also a basic stance in the standing practice. Holding the ball generates a roundness to the form. The standing practice generates energy. It is the starting movement and provides the energy for all the postures in the form.

Ward Off is the father. It is the basic posture of the form. It can generate to any of the other postures of the form. Practice using ward off and then create any of the other postures in the form. The energy that is generated in ward off migrates smoothly to those other postures.

Preparation

The initial steps in the preparation positions the feet with the inside arch in line with the center channel. This can be tested with a tool – a broomstick handle. Always have one in the studio. See the example of the measurement. This is not only an internal positioning where the energy of the channels is supported and add to the balance of the body but also provides a strong centered stance. The beginning and ending of the form is the only time a position will be taken that is 50/50 weighted. Of course the body will transition through a 50/50 position in every posture but the time spend is momentary and is an at risk position.

The body assumes it resting pose that is a strong and balanced stance but a deflated torso. This is done by allowing the two hip kua to close slightly allowing the upper body to tilt slightly forward an angle of 15 to 20 degrees of the spine. The shoulders are relaxed and the arms hang at the side. Refer back to the discussion on the Bend.

Now beginning the form, the hands go from palms facing the legs to a back of palm facing forward. This simple move has a grand effect. Simply turning the palms backwards allows the opening of the kua of the arm. (Armpit) This allows the shoulders to open and move outward away from the spine. The rib cage is then allowed to separate and will increase the pulmonary cavity and allow more room for the lungs. This simple move has now allowed the organs to move to their proper places, the lungs to expand and collapse with less effort and to allow the spine to raise up without the pressure from the shoulders. (See diagram)

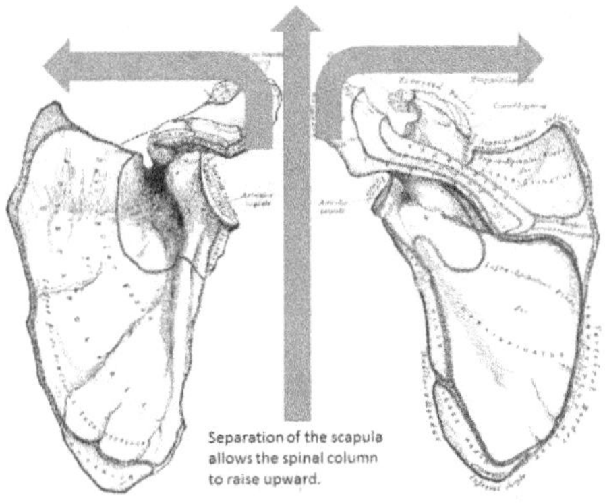

The thumb and first two fingers and the big toe are the initiators of the next action. The elbows and shoulders stay relaxed and follow the fingers to the raised position. The toe pushes down and twists inward sending energy up the spine. The fingers then relax and the elbows collapse inward. Here we see a broken wrist rather than maintaining the Fair Lady's wrist. When the elbows reach the apex of their circle the fingers reactivate and present an open palm – back to the Fair Lady's Wrist. This is commonly used as a block but a block can become a strike at any time. The fingers then relax and the hands drift down to a position at the sides of the hips while maintaining an open arm kua.

Hold the Ball

Often thought of as a transition posture, hold the ball has many martial functions as well as an opening of the joints posture. When holding the ball, the elbows should move away from the spine allowing the spine to rise, the rib cage to separate and to allow the flow of energy out of the arms to create a circle of energy. It is important to imagine holding a ball to get the upper and lower hands in the proper position. Practicing with a beach ball of appropriate size will teach how the lower hand and the upper hand need to be in the proper position to keep the ball from falling. The hands must also be at a distance to hold the ball without crowding the body or losing the ball when the hands are too far away.

Grasp the Sparrow's Tail

The next four movements are commonly combined into one name called Grasp the Sparrows Tail. These and all the next movements need to be practiced using the basic stances as the foundation of each movement as documented in the previous section under stances.

Ward Off

Ward Off is performed throughout the form whether it is the long or short form. A basic movement has very many applications. It comes from the previous application of Hold the ball. Two postures can be used. Only the yin hand is altered. Either that hand is at the same level of the warding hand just back from the arm or the hand is at a guarding position just inside of the hip. Both hands must maintain yang energy. The warding off arm should be relaxed and creating a circular shape with the hand in front of the center line of the body. If the hand is brought into the body, the hand should connect at the solar plexus. This makes a power connection as well as provides the strongest muscular connection. The hand should be relaxed but the fingers are straight and the wrist maintains Fair Lady's Wrist. Alternate postures incorporate left and right side as well as multiple stances. The normal posture is the bow stance with the lead foot and same side lead hand forward. The hands can be alternated to change from right ward off to left ward off without changing the stance. Ward off can also be from a back weighted stance providing another set of postures. There is even a ward off from the horse stance. Alternating arms and weight provides four more postures. Look at wave hands like clouds and see it in the middle of the movement. Grandmaster Chen uses ward off to get an understanding of changes of posture and stance outside of the form. This is a simple posture to start for understanding the variety of movement in the art.

Rollback

Roll back can be practiced three ways. In the Grandmaster Chen tradition, it becomes a chopping hand downward. Grandmaster Liang used the roll back "letting the robber in" allowing the opponent to commit as the player shifts to the back leg and then turns the waist to knock the opponent over. A third option is to use roll back in a rolling circle which provides for a throwing motion which starts at the forward position and completes on the rear leg. At no time should the front knee lock when moving into the back weighted position. This will lead to heaviness in the movement, heaviness into the next movement with the need to unlock the joint before initiating the movement and potential knee damage not only when doing the form but when using the movement in an application.

The movement starts with the A hand moving out to the SE corner ending at a 45-degree angle. The B hand moves across the body with the ending position across the body with the middle finger almost touching the elbow to connect the energy palm facing the body. The arms stay in this position as the weight is shifted to the back leg with the right arm slightly opening to allow a forward drop. When the weight is on the back leg, the root is established and then the action can be initiated. The waist turns with the right arm attached to the opponent's body and the left hand warding off the opponent's hands and the left palm turning upward as the waist turns. This upward motion helps break the root of the opponent as the right arm directs the opponent to the left side of the body and the right palm turns down.

In Grandmaster Chen system the movement is similar to start but the left palm is used to either grab and throw the opponent or to deflect a punch and the right hand is used to chop to the opponent most often to the shoulder or back of the neck.

The throw is when the right palm attaches to either the elbow, the shoulder or the opponents torso and the left hand grabs the opponents arm. The action is an upward movement following a circle down towards the ground. It is tricky to learn but performed smoothly by Master Yu.

Press

Press requires the elbows to be in the proper position to allow the connection to the body. The power comes from the body and not the hands. The pressing hand must connect to the arm at the wrist. If it connects to the hand, the weak spot is in the forward wrist. If it connects to the arm, the wrist of the front hand is at risk of a wrist lock. The connection should be the center of the palm (the laugong point) to the pivot point of the wrist.

Press is a connecting movement. Many players bring the hands together and then press outward turning it into a less powerful movement. The joining of hands should end this movement with the Mind directing the action of the press since the press is a Fa Jin movement and is used more often in this manner like a strike rather than a reinforced push. When playing Tui Shou the press should be played in an An manner, steady push to the partner's body.

Also in Grandmaster Chen system there is an alternative use with the forward hand, behind the opponent's head and the rear hand slamming into the head as a strike either as a fist but as most likely a palm strike.

Push

Push is easy. Think of hanging an old towel on the clothesline. Hold it with two fingers, thumb, and lift it over the line. Differentiate the substantial from the insubstantial. Never push equally with both hands. Alter the energy during the push to test the opponent's center and root. Push to and through the spine. Push the fullness to the emptiness. Remember that the thumbs are pushing in tacks.

Push should be a short and gentle movement. Move the opponent a quarter of an inch and break the root. Push hands is a practice for the martial applications of the art. A push can be used to knock an opponent over but often becomes a Fa Jin strike. A push to the opponent moving them only a few feet away puts the player in direct range of all the opponent's weapons. Using strength instead of gentleness, risks the loss of central equilibrium. Pushing equally with two hands is double weighted. If both hands are not yang, the energy will go from one side of the body to the other rather than into the opponent.

Single Whip

Single whip requires that the cocking of the hip is unseen. The hands stay at shoulder level in front of the body while the hip cocks. The fingers guide the movement across from the east to the north to the northwest. The hook hand forms as the right hand continues to circle to the chest staying round and soft until needed. Direct the energy to the hook until it reaches its ending point and then focus the attention to the left. The left hand raises up pivoting on the elbow until it is vertical. The pivot is in the elbow and guided by the shoulder. The left hand turns over palm away from body for a push or a strike.

Single Whip has many movements in the application. Also, learn to use the pivoting movements on the toe and heel as force is exerted.

Raise hands and step up

Open in a gesture of giving. Let the robber into the house before closing the trap. The palms are upward and the arms spread wide. The left foot is on its heel with the toe raised slightly. As the opponent advances, the arms turn into the center with the triggering of the trap. All three weapons are brought into play - two hands and a foot. The foot can be a kick or a sweep. If kicking, the movement has to stop at the opponent to retain central equilibrium. If sweeping the foot should skim the floor and encounter the opponent just below the ankle just as the hands apply force. The foot lays to the floor with only the width of a sheet of paper free under it to prevent the counter sweep.

Play the lute

This form is played in one of two ways. The first is the traditional movement with the hands locking the opponent from the side. The other is a Chin'na movement where the lock is vertical.

The opponent's arm is straight and within reach. The left arm is forward and the palm facing to the center. The right hand is closer to the chest and the palm faces to the center. The left hand goes to control the opponent's elbow. The right hand goes to the opponent's wrist. This is best used on a right arm that allows for an easy lock. Once connected both hand move towards the center of the opponent's arm locking arm. Hands in the form are slightly separated on the vertical. The left hand is at shoulder height with a slight bend. The right hand is closer to the chest near the solar plexus.

The second option changes the connection to the opponent. The left hand connects to the bottom of the elbow. The right hand connects to the wrist. The action is for the left arm to move upward and the right hand to push down on the wrist. This locks the arm into the shoulder. The end position is with the left hand palm up and the right hand palm down in the same positions as in the previous example.

If the opponent provides straightness, the lute player strings his instrument and captures the attack. One up and one down lock the attack. Only the player decides if the completion of the movement yields into a break or a throw. The energy adjustment of the rear foot at a right angle to the attack provides the energy from a strong root to control the attack.

Pull down to shoulder stroke

The pull is with the fingertips and guides the opponent's energy. It is not a tug but a continuous pull. The shoulder meets the opponent in a devastating move with little movement. If thrush forward, the player is using clumsy energy and will fall over losing central equilibrium. The spine becomes like an oak in the wind and accepts the energy as it comes from the opponent and reflects it back adding the player's energy. When considering the application of shoulder stroke the action is to guide the opponent as if they ran into a tree.

White Crane spreads wings

So many options as the bird stretch its wing from the body keeping the roundness in the length of the stretch. Arms and leg all move at once but none finishes at the same time. This adds to the variety. The Fair

Lady's wrist remains as the foot glides across the floor lightly touching the toe to the ground. The heel remains close to the ground. The right hand raises just to the eyebrow with the palm flat to the floor. The left hand moves down across the groin in a blocking movement and positions itself just at the side of the hip.

White Crane Spreads Both Wings

The movement, not seen in many of the later forms, can be substituted for the single wing or done as an additional movement as in Grandmaster Chen's long form. When performed as the primary movement both arms move the eyebrow position to complete the movement. If added to the form the raised arm lowers and the weight shifts to the unweighted foot. The now unweighted foot steps out as both arms raise to eye brow height.

Brush knee and push

Circles within circles this movement has all the options. From strikes, to throws, sweeps, kicks, all of Tai Chi Chuan is incorporated into Brush Knee. Learn it large but then hide all the options in the form until the opponent can see none. Loosen the hips for they need to pivot at each kua. Lightness of touch and leverage provides the energy for this movement. The left hand makes a large clockwise circle as the body pivots on the right hip turning to the side. The right hand also is making a circle in the same direction starting down when the left is rising. Then the hands reverse with the left going down and the right going up. The hands end with the left at the right hip and the right at the right ear. The left foot has stepped forward when the weight has shifted to the back right foot. The weight is shifted to the left foot as the body continues to turn back in a loading movement. When the weight has shifted to the left foot, the body turns to the left to a square position over the feet. The toes and fingers activate and the left hand clears the left knee. The right hand strikes or pushes the opponent's chest.

Let the opponent's movement provide the power to which he is struck or thrown. Find the strikes in the form. Transition from one side to the other provides movements that include throws and strikes. The opposite side is just a reverse of these movements. Shift the weight back and then turn out the front foot to move to the other side.

Catch tiger return to mountain

This movement starts with a shift to the left foot and a downward block with both hands protecting the groin and left leg. Only at that time does the player start the movement to the rear. The player turns using the left hip as the turning wheel. The right foot waits until the hips have opened the pelvic girdle and the body is focused to the southeast. The right foot then steps behind to a shoulder width position and touches heel down. As the weight is transferred into the right foot the right hand scoops down an around the knee ending palm facing forward at knee level and the left hand pushes shoulder height.

Needle at sea bottom

Raise the left and right hands to shoulder height in a compact circle. The left hand is placed on the right hand. Bend the spine as the hands come in. Then straighten it up and bend over at the kua to a comfortable level keeping the spine straight and strike or pull downward. Then raise back up with the spine curling up starting at the base of the spine ending with the spine upright.

Needle at Sea Bottom is done opposite of what many people do. The first part of the action is to relax the spine that causes a bending action. The spine then straightens as the player bends at the kua and directs the energy to a point on the floor just in from of the forward foot. Many people start with a straight spine and bend over to the bottom. This does not allow the proper energy to be exerted into the movement. The energy comes out of the foot up the back and down the arm. A straight back only can manage the flow of energy. This movement is a locking techniques or a strike.

Apparent Closing Up

Apparent Closing Up is a wide opening to a closing movement. Apparent Closing Up is seen in two formats in the long form. The first is when one arm has extended and the other opens out to the side presenting the opponent a wide open target. The second is when both arms open out from the body and then close to the cross hands stance. This is a large movement and should be an opening of the shoulders and arms and then the pulling together into a crossed hand stance in front of the body but still a full rounded body and arms. The arms are rounded like holding a small ball in front of the body. The hands are activated with the finger in a straight position. There are numerous hidden techniques in this simple movement and they will be covered in another volume. For now the practice is a great rounded opening and a wide circular motion to a comfortable open cross hands position palms at chest height facing in.

Cross hands

See Apparent Closing up above for the preparation for this posture. Also called sealing up in many forms. This is referencing the movement after Deflect and Punch where one arm is extended and then the movement into Cross Hands. Cross hands needs to be practice in many postures since it is part of many postures though seldom seen.

Now the action. The weight shifts to the left leg as the arms open. The right arm stays as the body turns and the left arm swings across until the body is open. Both hands then circle down, come up in front of the body, and create a cross. In this simple movement, there are many variables and applications.

Withdraw and Push

The left hand wraps under the elbow wiping the right arm and across the wrist when both hands spread out and return with a double-handed push. Remember that in all pushes there is a yin and yang balance with one hand pushing more than the other does. This creates a twisting movement in the opponent's body and allows for the breaking of the root.

Wave hands like clouds

The right Hand is at shoulder height with the palm facing the body. The left arm is at waist height with the palm upwards. Both arms are rounded. The stance is a horse stance with the distance varying with the step but the weight always on one side. The weight is on the right leg. The waist turns the torso to the right as the right hand stays in its position in regards to the body. The left hand strikes out to the right under the right arm. The arms shift position with the left hand up and the right hand down palms also changing. The left foot steps out the left just longer than shoulder height. The body then starts shifting the weight to the left leg and the body turns back to center. When all the weight is on the left leg and the waist is centered, the waist turns with the left arm blocking and the right hand striking to the opponent's lower body. The repeat movement is for the right leg to step in to a stance inside the shoulder width and the same actions going to the right side. This can be repeated any number of times.

Snake creeps down

The snake strikes when not expected.

The left hand strikes forward as right foot turns out and the weight shifts back. The left hand retreats to the chest and then strikes directly downward ending in the center of the body as the back follows. The back does not bend going down but straightens on the strike. The waist turns as the left hand continues to the extended left leg and strikes again. See the reverse of the movement. Not all movements are as they appear. This movement can also use the energy to throw the opponent backward.

High Pat Horse

The hands start at the center line. The left hand is extending to the front at chest height. The right fingers start at the inside elbow of the left arm and slide out to the end of the arm and then continue to a high shoulder level position in front of the body with the palm in opposition – left palm is up and right palm is down. The right foot moves into the position next to the left foot on the initial movement. The weight shifts to the right leg and the left leg steps out to the toe providing for a kick.

Golden cock stands on one leg

Think of taking giant steps. When on the left side, bend the back and close the kua to get the connection to the energy and then straighten the back drawing the left foot upward with the back. The left hands follows the foot and continues upward to a bent position with the tiger mouth open and the player looking through the tiger's mouth. The left hand then retreats to the inside as you step down to the heel of the left foot rolling into the front of the foot. The back bends at the kua to gain the connection to the energy. When all the weight is shifted to the left foot, the right foot is raised with the right hand following and continuing up to the tiger mouth in front of the eyes. The knee is one of the weapons of this movement. The energy is focused on the foot to insure that the energy cycle is complete.

Separate foot

Remember the rollbacks in the transitions of this movement. Snap the chopsticks when kicking. The kick does not come from the kicking leg but from the base leg otherwise it is just a Li or muscle powered kick. Practice these kicks individually as a way of development the whole body kick rather than a leg action.

Turn and kick with heel

The body closes with the arms withdrawing to the chest and the foot raised up from the floor but located just in front of the opposite knee. The kua of the right hip closes and the back bends to gain the energy as the body turns slightly to the right. The body spins on the right heel 180 degrees to the left. The power is from the right hip and can use the left foot as an added energy source. The left leg stays close to the body as it spins with the left arm staying on the outside coming up to the wrist of the right hand with both hands open. This can also be done as a wiping movement with the left hand wiping from the right elbow out to the right wrist. The back bends and the kua closes making the connection to the energy source. The left leg kicks outward striking with the heel as the body straightens. The energy comes from the rooted foot and not from the snapping of the leg.

Turn to sweep the lotus

The internal body cocks by loosening the right hip leaving the arms in their current position. This prevents telegraphing the next movement. It also provides an internal twist exercising the thorax and supporting muscles and organs. The spin is performed, as a skater would execute a fast movement with the arms in and the leg close to the body providing a faster spin. The first two nails are released and the spin is on the heel or third nail. This allows a weighted turn without risking an injury to the knee.

An alternative turn justifiably titled by Grandmaster Liang is the old man's turn. This involves a three step turn. As the waist turns to the back, the unweighted leg steps down towards the back. The weight is shifted to that foot and the other foot follows stepping down and away forming an L. Continuing the turn the weight shifts and the unweighted foot steps to a pigeon toe position and the weight transfers again. This completes the turn. This is done in slow motion allowing seniors to make this turn without risk of injury or falling. This also has interesting application implications that will be discussed in the next volume.

Sweeping the Lotus is performed by cocking the body but leaving the hands in position. Again, do not broadcast the next action. The leg raises up and across as the body turns while the hands stay in position. Do not worry about the hands touching the toes. This can cause the player to bend forward completing the movement with a bent back. The back should be, as the classics say, straight and the head upright. Allowing the hands to brush across the knees will complete this movement and hold to the principles of Tai Chi Chuan and at the same time provides a more valid application of this movement. Most people assume that the hands must brush the foot as the foot is the lotus but the lotus is an attacking structure of the body in this movement. Full description of the use of this kick is in the San Shou Volume.

Parting Wild Horse's Mane

Parting the Mane is a long smooth motion. The movement starts with both hands at the center line. The right hand scoops palm up and rides out through the center line while the left hand palm down moves down and back to the left hip. This movement has the smoothness of drawing silk. The torso starts with a slight bend and opens to provide full energy to the movement. There is an open feeling to the upper body. The arms though extended maintain an indication of roundness. Do not over extend on each of the movements. Do not straighten the arms.

Diagonal flying

This movement can be an extremely long and open movement. It works in that manner and helps to stretch the body. In practice, the movement should be played much shorter and the movement of the extended arm is pivoting at the elbow rather than the shoulder. In action, this keeps the attacking arm from being at risk of a lock and the pivot point is closer to the player's body. It also allows the circle of attack to be more precise and directed at turning the opponent off their root in a twisting manner.

Repulse monkey

Repulse Monkey is not only a backward movement away from the opponent but also includes rearward attack options. Therefore, the focus needs to be on completeness of the movements in both directions. The rearward hand should not break the back.[36] The body turns on the alternate hip and the action hip makes the foot move backwards. Do not lift the foot to step. The hip makes the leg move backwards. The toe touches down and assures the footing. The weight is shifted into the foot and a root is obtained. Once the root is established, the hand pulls downward and the other hand attacks forward.

Fair lady works the shuttle 4 corners

Fair Lady finds all four corners. The movement is easy but the turns are difficult. The basic movements of Fair Lady are below. As the front foot steps out, the opposite hand blocks circularly backward at ear level. The front arm raises lifting the opponent up and opening their body to attack. The weight shifts to the forward foot and the opposite hand strikes the opponent with the palm.

The turns are difficult due to the large angles in two of them. The diagram below shows how to get from corner to corner.

Remember the rollbacks throughout each of these movements that come as part of the body turning. The hands weave in a pattern of threes – deflect back, raise up and strike out. Step behind and not out while making the transitions. There is one hand position as seen below that preps the movements of each Lady. It is also valuable throughout the Tai Chi Chuan applications. Practice it and learn its options.

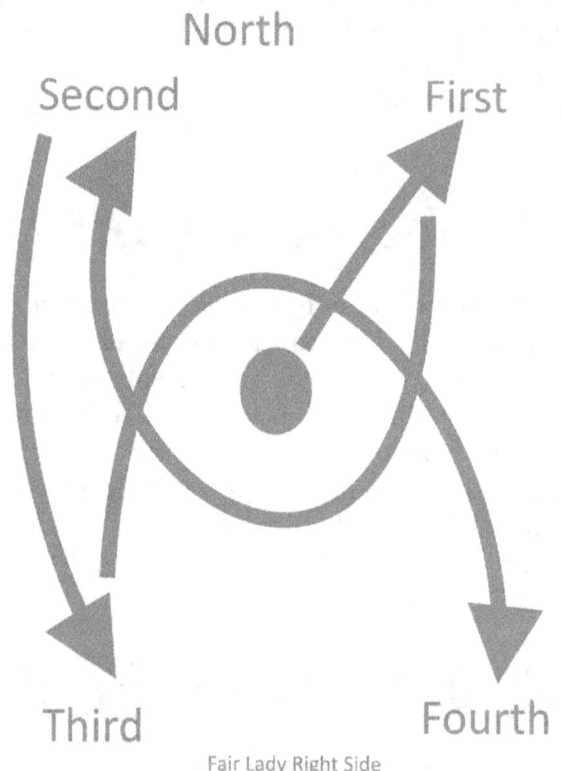

Fair Lady Right Side

Fan penetrates back

Do not look at the instructor. Fan penetrates the back is a square posture with the body and hips square to the footing foundation. Players have a habit of looking at the instructor to see if they are doing the form correctly and end up with a sideways posture. The application resembles the jab in boxing. The forward hand strikes out with the fingers or a fist and the rear hand protects the head.

Deflect, Parry and Punch

There are two ways of doing this posture. The traditional is to incorporate the movements as in the name. The right hand in a fist and the left hand with an open palm deflects a punch down and to the player's right side. The opponent then swing the deflect arm around to hit to the players left side of the head. The player brings up the left hand to parry the swinging punch of the opponent. The player then punches to the center of the opponent with the right hand in a fist.

The second option is more aggressive. The player deflects an attack with the right hand in a loose fist down and to the right and immediately strikes forward and down with the left hand in a chopping strike and then follows it with the right fist to the opponents center.

In either format the left hand and arm provides a running block for any action of the opponent on the players left side and opens up a path for the attack to the center with the right fist.

Brush knee and strike downward

This is a modified brush knee with the body turning to the right as the player steps forward heel to toe with the left leg. The weight shifts to the left leg. The left hand goes to the right side and sweeps down to the left knee in a brushing movement. The right hand holds a loose fist and strikes down to the opponent's groin just after the left hand brushes the knee. The bend is at the waist (Kua) not bending the back.

Bend Bow and Shoot the Tiger

This is a retreating attack. The player steps to the side with the right foot. The weight shifts to the right leg. The hands retreat backward in a lowering circle coming back towards the body. The two fist stay in alignment with the tiger mouths facing each other. The circle continues and attacks the opponent both high and low.

Twin peaks pierce ears

This is a perfect example of the multiple weapon attack of Tai Chi Chuan. An attack from the knee can turn to a front kick and the two weapons of the hands attack at once to the temples. When attacking with multiple weapons the balance of yang in each attacking weapon is different. One always leads. As in a push, you only push with one hand the other is reinforcing the attack and prepared to assist in the application of force.

Chop and strike to the groin

The left foot turns out to the left just short of 90 degrees. The left hand forms an open palm and the right hand makes a fist. The right foot steps close to the heel of the left foot forming a v shape. The right hand goes to the groin as the left hand goes to the left shoulder. The right circles up to the shoulder height as the right foot raises. The right foot steps out to the heel. The left hand circles out and chops in front of the body as the right hand also circling closer to the chest and deflects down. The left leg steps forward with the left hand strike. The weight shifts to the left leg. The left hand brushes the left knee and the right hand strikes down toward the opponent's groin.

Chop with fist right penetrating hand

Withdraw into the circle allowing the hands to find their circle in front of the body. The hands stay open and free during their loop with a weight shift to the right leg and turn the body. Shift the weight back to the left as the right leg steps out as the chop comes off the back foot (left). Plant the root before initiating the chop that is a flipping action striking with the first and second knuckles of the right hand. The left hand follows with an open palm and a push down. The weight shifts to the right foot. The left leg steps forward to the heel. The left hand stays energized as the weight shifts to the new front leg and the right hand strikes outward with the fingers over the left arm.

Chop with Fist

The older form of the Yang Long Form included the Chop back fist move at the ending of all three sections. This was the use of a long back fist movement. It is a powerful movement making use of not only the impact of the internal energy but the use of a large attacking circle. There are two versions used. The fist at the ending of the first section is a cross-body back fist. The left leg is forward and weighted. The right hand starts at the left hip and circles up and then down to the point of impact. The left hand is used to clear the path starting at the right elbow and moving to the left hip.

The second method used in section two and three is a similar movement. The right foot steps out to the corner and assumes the weight. The hand movements are the same. This is a right chop from a right weighted side. Many may argue that this is double weighted. The weight is on the right side but single weighted into the right leg. See the discussion on use of the tools of the body and the weight distribution.

Beat Tiger

Beat Tiger is a retreating posture only to draw the opponent in to be met with the force of the two fists. The player steps back and allows the arms to drop providing the opponent an opening. As the opponent prepares their counter by moving towards the body, the player's arms come back up and meet the opponent. In the form the posture is back weighted but the same counter attack can be made with the weight shifting forward with a two handed attack. Remember that always one hand is the leader in an attack – both hands are not equally powered otherwise you are double weighted.

Fist under elbow

The left arm circles behind the left hip crosses the chest back to the left side with the tiger's mouth open and away from the body. This can be a strike, a block, or a grab. The right hand forms a loose fist directly under the left elbow and the left leg steps out to the heel with the toe slightly off the ground. Do not break the back[37] when reaching with the left arm.

Step back to ride the tiger

The step back avoids an attack and provides a counter attack. The hands descend staying crossed but open to catch the attack. The back stays straight but the body bends at the kua to reach the attack. The forward hand brushes the attack away or catches a late kick and the rear hand comes up to the side of the head palm forward used as a block or a strike with either a chop or a tiger mouth fist.

Step up to seven stars

Upon moving forward, the hands take the lead blocking a downward attack. The forward hand when attacked is a blocking hand and moves much slower than the rear hand. The fists stay open and soft using the root energy rather than arm strength. In striking, the tiger mouth is the impact point. In defensive situation, the forward hand is again the blocking hand and the rear hand charges in to provide support. The leg is a follower in this movement. It comes up to provide a sweep or kick after the completion of the hand maneuvers. The leg comes forward as the hands connect with the heel on the floor and the toe raised just off the floor. Raising the toe more draws energy into the leg and it is not relaxed and the raised toe draws energy back toward the body destabilizing this position.

Turn and Chop with Fist

There are a number of turns involving chops in the form. They provide transition from one direction to another but it is very valuable to understand their use. The old classics discuss this posture as starting with an elbow strike and then surprise the opponent with a blossoming fist. That is not the only surprise in this movement. The body starts facing one direction. The weight shifts to the right leg. The hands rotate in a circle up and around coming back to the body. The right hand is at the left hip as is the left hand – the right to the center. The left foot turns in as the hands circle and then when pointing towards the new direction the weight shifts to the left leg. The right leg is unweighted.

There are two options at this time. The right leg can step back with the ending of the circle. This protects the right leg or prepares for use of the right foot. The feet would be close together with the weight remaining on the left leg. The right leg then steps out and assumes the weight. The arms again circle with the right hand becoming a back fist and the left hand a following chop. The right hand lowers to the right hip and the left hand stays in a protective position at shoulder height.

The other option is for the right leg to stay and assume the weight as the arms start their new circle out. The right back fist strikes out and comes back to the hip as the left remains in a protective position. The reasons and options in this movement are discussed in the next volume.

White Snake Puts out its tongue

This movement is performed exacting as the previous discussed movement. The ending changes with a finger strike. The fist opens palm up and the fingers open to strike the opponent. The left hand assumes a position at the right elbow palm down remaining out as the right hand retreats to the right hip. Again, the right foot remains or it is pulled back during the move. Since this is a snake strike, the step back is reminiscent of a snake striking.

Torso Flung Fist

Not seen in all forms, this is one of the basic punches used in Tai Ch'i Chuan. It is located in older versions of the form just before deflect parry and punch. The old yang version of Grandmaster Liang has the long chops in this location but he included this punch in the Tai Ch'i Chuan Dance. This is a powerful punch using the twisting of the waist to power the fist. The right hand in a loose fist goes to the left hip palm down and the left hand raises up few inches above the fist with an open palm facing down. The right foot moves into a position just in front of the left rooted foot toe only on the ground. The waist is turned to the left as the right fist moves to the hip. The right fist moves across the body as the right foot steps out to the front and right of the body with the turning back of the waist. The fist turns into a standing fist and hits the opponent from the left rooted foot. The left hand moves out and away to the left front of the body.

Yang Style Tai Chi Chuan Forms

The Tai Chi Chuan form has many styles and forms. The major styles are Chen, Wu, and Yang with many other styles practiced. Each of these styles has variations depending upon the lineage and the teacher. The focus here is on the Grandmaster Chen's Yang style. Even the Yang style has many different variations. The long Yang form is practiced by many of the second-generation players from the Professor's lineage. Just to mention a few, Grandmaster Liang did a version of the long form and did not teach any short versions. Master Lo and Master Yu both taught long form. All three of these teachers taught the same basic form but each was different. Each teacher focuses on different techniques and stances. Since there has been a formalized competition, we have now seen many new varieties of the form usually a lessening of the number of movements such as the 8, 13, 16, and 24-movement form.

Many people try to learn all of these forms. It is not necessary but will not hurt you. The Professor taught the short form. Grandmaster Chen primarily teaches his short form but teaches his long form once a year at his studio. Grandmaster Liang only taught the long form. All were involved with the background techniques that make up the Tai Chi Chuan art. The important part of Tai Chi Chuan is to learn the basic principles and apply them to your form whether it is a long form or a short form. Tai Chi Chuan started with only the 13 original movements. Grandmaster Liang always said that even the long form was not long enough to get the Ch'i flowing. He advocated the approach of Right - Left - Right when practicing - meaning to do the form on both sides

There is a history to the form. Originally, Tai Chi Chuan was taught one movement at a time. The student would study that movement until the master decided he understood the movement. This could be studying single whip for years. Since there were few books due to cost and many people were illiterate the way to remember the movements as the student progressed was to link them together into a form. This is a very plausible story and is a valid reason for generating forms. Now it is just history for most people but a few learned teachers have remembered the need to understand the movement and teach in addition to the form the study of the applications. Always remember that a movement does not necessarily relate to the movement before or after it. When doing the form be aware that it is easy to fall into the habit of flowing from one move to the next. The form needs definition and each movement needs a beginning and an end. That ending may only be the internal change in energy but that change (think yin to yang) must be there.

It is the understanding of the form that is important and not the order. If you want to practice by learning different forms, it is up to you. It is important to stay within your style until you understand the complexity and intricate movements of your form to get the most out of your practice. Understanding the different styles and their variations is important to knowing your own style but as one teacher said, do not mix your milk and orange juice in the morning.

The Form Lists

Eight Movement Form

Commencing form

Repulse Monkey Right, left;

Grasp Sparrow's Tail: ward off, rollback,press, push

Wave Hands Like Clouds Left 3 times

Fair Lady Works Shuttles Left and right

Golden Cock Stands One Leg Right and Left

Brush Knees and Twist Step Left and Right

Apparent Closing Up

Yang Tai Chi Chuan 13 Movement Form

Preparation

Beginning Posture

Wave Hands like Clouds

Single Whip

Fist under Elbow

White Crane Spreads its Wings

Left Brush Knee

Hands Play the Lute

High Pat on Horse with Palm Thrust

Turn Body and Chop with Fist

Step Forward, Parry and Punch

Grasp the Bird's Tail

Cross Hands

Closing

Yang Tai Chi Chuan 16 Movement Form

Preparation Form

Wave Hands like Clouds (1)

Single Whip

Fist under Elbow

White Crane Spreads its Wings

Left Brush Knee and Push

Hand Plays the Lute

Step Back and Repulse the Monkey

Left Strike Tiger

Parting Wild Horse's Mane

Step Forward and Punch Downward

Turn Body and White Snake Spits out Tongue

Step Forward, Parry, Block, and Punch

Step Forward and Grasp the Bird's tail

Cross Hands

Closing

Tai Chi 24 Form (Beijing Form)

Beginning

Part the Wild Horse's Mane (Left and Right)

White Crane Spreads Its Wings

Brush Knee and Step Forward (Left and Right)

Playing the Lute

Step Back and Repulse Monkey (Left and Right)

Left Grasp Sparrow's Tail (Ward Off Rollback, Press, and Push)

Right Grasp Sparrow's Tail

Single Whip

Wave Hands Like Clouds

Single Whip

High Pat on Horse

Separate Left Foot

Separate Right Foot

Strike to Ears with Both Fists

Turn Body and Kick with Left Heel

Left Golden Rooster Stands on One Leg

Right Golden Rooster Stands on One Leg

Fair Lady Works with Shuttles

Needle at Sea Bottom

Fan Through Back

Turn Body, Deflect, Parry, and Punch

Apparent Close Up

Cross Hands

Closing

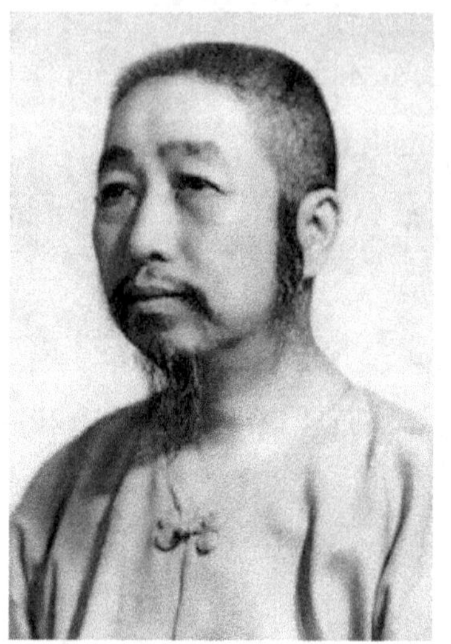

Cheng Man Ching's 37 Movements

Part 1

Preparation

Beginning

Ward Off Left

Ward Off Right

Roll Back

Press

Push

Single Whip

Raise Hands

Wave Hands like Clouds Right

Single Whip

Snake Creeps Down

Golden Cock Stands on One Leg, Right

Golden Cock Stands on One Leg, Left

Separation of the Right Foot

Separation of the Left Foot

Turn Body and Kick with Heel

Brush Knee, Left

Brush Knee, Right

Step Forward and Punch

Grasping the Sparrow's Tail*

Single Whip

Fair Lady Weaves at the Shuttle

Fair Lady Weaves at the Shuttle

Fair Lady Weaves at the Shuttle

Fair Lady Weaves at the Shuttle

Grasping the Sparrow's Tail*

Single Whip

Snake Creeps Down

Step Up to Seven Stars

Retreat to Ride Tiger

Turn Body Sweep Lotus Leg

Bend Bow Shoot Tiger

Step up, block, parry, and punch

Apparent Close-up, Cross Hands

Close

* The movements of press, push and roll back are frequently referred to as "Grasp the Sparrow's tail" and are frequently counted as one movement.

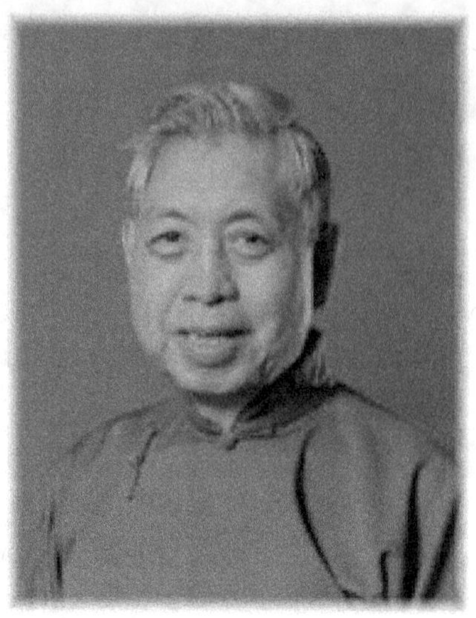

William Chen 60 Movements

Note that this form stays very close to that of the Professor's.

Part 1

1. Preparation

2. Beginning Posture

3. Ward Off Left

4. Ward Off Right

5. Rollback

6. Press

7. Push

8. Single Whip

9. Raise Hands and Step Up

10.   Pull Down to Shoulder Stroke

31.	Snake Creeps Down

32.	Golden Cock Stands On One Leg Right Side

33.	Golden Cock Stands On One Leg Left Side

34.	Separate Right Foot

35.	Separate Left Foot

36.	Turn and Kick with Heel

37.	Brush Knee and Strike Downward

38.	Twin Peaks Pierce Ears

39.	Rollback

40.	Press

41.	Push

42.	Single Whip

43.	Fair Lady Works the Shuttle

44.	Fair Lady Works the Shuttle

45.	Fair Lady Works the Shuttle

46.	Fair Lady Works the Shuttle

47.	Left Ward Off

48.	Right Ward Off

49.	Rollback

50.	Press

51.	Push

William Chen Long Form

Part 1

1. Preparation
2. Beginning Posture
3. Left Ward Off
4. Right Ward Off
5. Roll Away
6. Press
7. Push
8. Single Whip
9. Raise Hands
10. White Crane Spreads It's Wings
11. Brush Knee and Twist Step Left
12. Brush Knee and Twist Step Right
13. Brush Knee and Twist Step Left
14. Play the Fiddle
15. Step-up, Strike, Parry and Punch
16. Apparent Close –up
17. Cross Hands

Part 2

18. Carry Tiger to the Mountain
19. Roll away
20. Press
21. Push
22. Diagonal Single Whip

23.	Fist under Elbow
24.	Step back Repulse Monkey Right
25.	Step back Repulse Monkey Left
26.	Step back Repulse Monkey Right
27.	Diagonal Flying
28.	Raise Hands
29.	White Crane Spreads it's Wings
30.	White Crane Spreads both Wings[38]
31.	Brush Knee and Twist Step Left
32.	Needle at Sea Bottom
33.	Fan through Back
34.	Turn and Hit with Back Fist
35.	Step-up, Strike, Parry and Punch
36.	Step up and Ward off Right
37.	Roll Away
38.	Press
39.	Push
40.	Single Whip
41.	Wave Hands like Clouds Left
42.	Wave Hands like Clouds Right
43.	Wave Hands like Clouds Left
44.	Single Whip
45.	High Pat Horse Right
46.	Kick with Right Toe
47.	High Pat Horse Left
48.	Kick with Left Toe

10.	Ward Off Left
11.	Ward Off Right
12.	Roll Away
13.	Press
14.	Push
15.	Single Whip
16.	Fair Lady Works the Shuttle (4 Corners)
17.	Ward Off Left
18.	Ward Off Right
19.	Roll Away
20.	Press
21.	Push
22.	Single Whip
23.	Wave Hands like Clouds Left
24.	Wave Hands like Clouds Right
25.	Wave Hands like Clouds Left
26.	Single Whip
27.	Snake Creeps Down
28.	Golden Cock Stands on One Leg Right
29.	Golden Cock Stands on One Leg Left
30.	Step Back and Repulse Monkey Right
31.	Step Back and Repulse Monkey Left
32.	Step Back and Repulse Monkey Right
33.	Slanting Flying
34.	Raise Hands
35.	White Stork spreads It's Wings

36.   Brush Knee and Twist Step Left

37.   Needle at Sea Bottom

38.   Fan through Back

39.   White Snake Puts Out Its Tongue.

40.   Step-up, Strike, Parry and Punch

41.   Step up and Ward off Right

42.   Roll Away

43.   Press

44.   Push

45.   Single Whip

46.   Wave Hands like Clouds Left

47.   Wave Hands like Clouds Right

48.   Wave Hands like Clouds Left

49.   Single Whip

50.   High Pat the Horse and Strike with Fingers

51.   Turn and Kick with Right Sole

52.   Brush Knee and Twist Step Right

53.   Step up and Punch at Groin

54.   Step up and Ward off Right

55.   Roll Away

56.   Press

57.   Push

58.   Single Whip

59.   Snake Creeps Down

60.   Step Up to Form Seven Stars

61.   Step Back to Ride Tiger

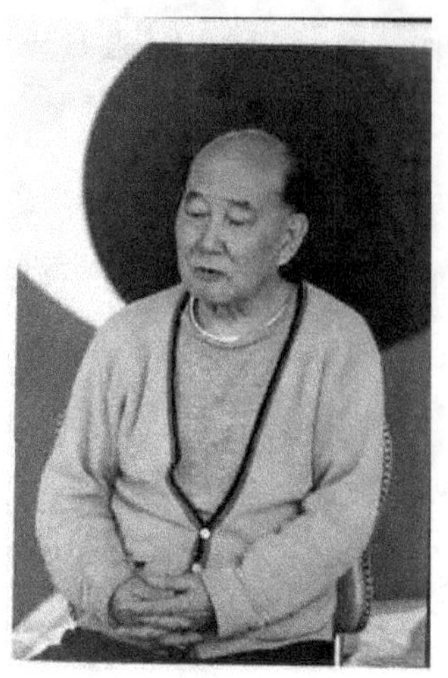

T. T. Liang Long Form

Part 1

1. Preparation

2. Beginning Posture

3. Left Ward Off

4. Right Ward Off

5. Roll Back

6. Press

7. Push

8. Single Whip

9. Raise Hands

10.   White Crane Spreads It's Wings

11.   Brush Knee and Twist Step Left

12.   Brush Knee and Twist Step Right

13.   Brush Knee and Twist Step Left

14.   Play the Flute

15.	Brush Knee and Twist Step Left
16.	Chop with Right Fist
17.	Step-up, Parry and Punch
18.	Apparent Closing –up
19.	Cross Hands

Part 2

18.	Carry Tiger and Return to the Mountain
19.	Roll back
20.	Press
21.	Push
22.	Diagonal Single Whip
23.	Fist under Elbow
24.	Step back Repulse Monkey Right
25.	Step back Repulse Monkey Left
26.	Step back Repulse Monkey Right
27.	Step back Repulse Monkey Left
28.	Step back Repulse Monkey Right
29.	Diagonal Flying
30.	Raise Hands
31.	White Crane Spreads it's Wings
32.	Brush Knee and Twist Step Left
33.	Needle at Sea Bottom
34.	Fan through Back
35.	Turn and Chop with Fist
36.	Step-up, Parry and Punch
37.	Step up and Ward off Right

38.   Roll back

39.   Press

40.   Push

41.   Single Whip

42.   Wave Hands like Clouds Left

43.   Wave Hands like Clouds Right

44.   Wave Hands like Clouds Left

45.   Wave Hands like Clouds Right

46.   Wave Hands like Clouds Left

47.   Single Whip

48.   High Pat Horse Right

49.   Kick with Right Toe

50.   Kick with Left Toe

51.   Turn and Kick with Sole

52.   Brush Knee and Twist Step Left

53.   Brush Knee and Twist Step Right

54.   Step Up and Punch Downward

55.   Turn and Chop with Fist

56.   Step-up, Parry and Punch

57.   Kick with Right Sole

58.   Beat the Tiger at Right

59.   Beat the Tiger at Left

60.   Kick with Right Heel

61.   Twin Peaks Pierce the Ears

62.   Kick with Left Heel

63.   Turn around and Kick with Right Heel

39.	Single Whip
40.	Wave Hands like Clouds Left
41.	Wave Hands like Clouds Right
42.	Wave Hands like Clouds Left
43.	Single Whip
44.	Snake Creeps Down
45.	Golden Cock Stands on One Leg Right
46.	Golden Cock Stands on One Leg Left
47.	Step Back and Repulse Monkey Right
48.	Step Back and Repulse Monkey Left
49.	Step Back and Repulse Monkey Right
50.	Diagonal Flying
51.	Raise Hands
52.	White Stork spreads It's Wings
53.	Brush Knee and Twist Step Left
54.	Needle at Sea Bottom
55.	Fan through Back
56.	White Snake Puts Out Its Tongue.
57.	Step-up, Parry and Punch
58.	Step up and Ward off Right
59.	Roll back
60.	Press
61.	Push
62.	Single Whip
63.	Wave Hands like Clouds Left
64.	Wave Hands like Clouds Right

65.	Wave Hands like Clouds Left
66.	Single Whip
67.	High Pat the Horse
68.	Left Piercing Hand
69.	Turn and Kick with Right Sole
70.	Brush Knee and Twist Step Right
71.	Step up and Punch at Groin
72.	Step up and Ward off Right
73.	Roll back
74.	Press
75.	Push
76.	Single Whip
77.	Snake Creeps Down
78.	Step Up to Form Seven Stars
79.	Step Back to Ride Tiger
80.	Turn Around Sweep the Lotus
81.	Bend the Bow and Shoot the Tiger
82.	Cross Body Chop with Fist
83.	Step-up, Parry and Punch
84.	Apparent Closing Up
85.	Cross Hands

Repetitive Movements

Throughout the forms, there are movements that are used either to extend the form and practice or to make a change from one application or direction to another. Single Whip is a common transitive movement for changing directions. Wave Hands, Repulse Monkey, Parting Wild Horse's

Mane, and Brush Knee are traveling movements – getting to another point in the form. It can be an easy practice to add more repetitions in these areas to add to any of the forms. If added going one direction, balance out the set by repeating another transitive movement going the opposite direction to end at your beginning posture. It will add to the interest of playing the form.

The lists of transitive and traveling movements are below. Tai Chi Players practice the form as often as possible. If the need for time is pressing, these transitive movements can be cut down, as seen in short forms, to a single movement or if time is available their number is increased.

Transitive Movements

Single Whip

Turn and Chop with Fist

Separate Hands

Traveling Movements

Brush Knee

Repulse Monkey

Wave Hands like Clouds

Parting Wild Horse's Mane

Left and Right

There is some controversy on the balance of Tai Chi Chuan and if the form should be done on both sides. Grandmaster Liang said that a round of Tai Chi Chuan was right, left and right sides. Grandmaster Chen teaches that both sides are done though he lets the player work on the left side of the form outside of class.

The Professor was noted as saying that the form was balanced when doing it on the right side and the left side was not good. He referenced the meridians as being impacted. He was also dedicated to reducing the form to its basic components. It may have been in his effort to reduce the learning process and compel people to continue to do the form that he simplified the form to only the right side.

Practicing the form, the left side is a weaker side since it is not practiced as often. In Tai Chi Chuan as a martial art, there is no room in fighting for the single sided fighter. Modern boxing has this problem since they focus only on the boxer's dominant side. Good fighters learn to be switch hitters. Everyone has a dominant hand but must feel comfortable with the opposite side.

Doing the form on both, the sides will balance out the body. Take one movement and do it on the right side. Then do it on the left side. You will find that it is working a different set on body parts. The art of Tai Chi Chuan is to balance out the body and to create the greatest flow of energy. Success at this will gain the greatest health benefits. Many people have back issues. Most back issues are one sided. A balanced system heals those issues. Focusing on doing one movement to work on the injury will not support the balancing of the body. One side of the form limits the tools to work on an injury.

Many people have learned both sides in both the form and weapon sets. This is very beneficial since it balances out the weight of the weapon as well as the body. Doing the left side of any single weapon set is very difficult but playing with double weapons will help. This cannot be done with a staff or spear but functions very well with the sword, knife, or cane. The staff and the spear are held with both hands playing on both sides.

So in conclusion do not limit your growth. Practice on both sides that which you can. Getting to the stage of the Professor, then the player can decide if the meridians are being impacted. Also, always go to a good quality Traditional Chinese Medicine doctor quarterly for the seasonal checkups.

Both Sides Now

One way to add variety to the practice of Tai Chi Chuan is to learn not only the long form and short form but to learn the left side of forms. Most other teachers recommend this - Grandmaster Liang and Grandmaster Chen both doing both sides. After learning the opposite side, then begin to play with the forms. Add different parts of the forms together to make up a new form. It breaks up the form increasing focus of the form and the side. It a very valuable tool to understand every movement of the form as well as developing the number of engrams in the mind.

Using three forms from this volume[39] the mix can be created by combining each part in different orders.

Yang[40] Long Section 1 Right Side = A

Yang Long Section 2 Right Side = B

Yang Long Section 3 Right Side = C

Yang Long Section 1 Left Side = D

Yang Long Section 2 Left Side = E

Yang Long Section 3 Left Side = F

Wm Chen Short Form Section 1 Right Side = G

Wm Chen Short Form Section 2 Right Side = H

Wm Chen Short Form Section 1 Left Side = I

Wm Chen Short Form Section 2 Left Side = J

Professor's Cheng Form Section 1 Right Side = K

Professor's Cheng Form Section 2 Right Side = L

Professor's Cheng Form Section 1 Left Side = M (No Disrespect Intended Professor)

Professor's Cheng Form Section 2 Left Side = N

That provides fourteen different sets to combine. Only three sections in a practice will provide 364 combinations - enough to keep practice from getting boring! Practice the normal morning and nightly rounds. Then create a practice form by adding a mix of the segments to create a practice form for a training session. Although this seems a lot, it does not take much time. As a couple of example are listed below:

K + L + G + H + A + B + C (Professor's Cheng Form - Wm Chen 60 Moves - Yang Long Form)

A + H + N (Yang Long Section 1 Right Side - Wm Chen Short

Form Section 2 Right Side- Professor's Form Section 2 Left Side)

A + D + G (Yang Long Section 1 Right Side + Yang Long Section 1 Left Side + Wm Chen Short Form Section 1 Right Side)

You get the idea. It will give you some new life to your practice and give you a chance to keep all your forms sharp.

Tui Shou and San Shou

Tui Shou – pushing hands and San Shou – free fighting are such involved topics that they will be discussed in their dedicated volumes. Single Circling Hands, a beginning exercise in Tui Shou, will be discussed so that the player can start to learn how to play with another partner.

Single Circling Hands is played with two people joining one arm at the wrist and circling the hands horizontally between each player to learn the basics of Tai Chuan. Each player stands in a bow stance same leg forward. The front foot of each player is on the inside of the opponent's foot. Placement isn't critical since it varies once the exercises move into advanced stages. Each player assumes ward off – start with the right hand and right foot forward. The left hand is held at the side hip level. One player, A, will start by shifting the weight into the front leg and circling the right arm towards the other player's body, B. A's attack should be in a straight direction towards B's body. B presents their right ward off and shifts the weight back as A advances and then turns the waist to the right to direct the attack away from the body. A retreats with the right becoming a ward off as B attacks. B tries to move straight into A's body but A's ward off moves back as the weight is shifted to the back leg and then A turns to the right to redirect the attack away. This pattern continues training the players in methods of weight shifting, staying attached and circular movements. Once the players become familiar with the movements, the legs can be changed and the arms can be changed making four methods of this form. Once reaching this stage the attacks can change at level and hand posture used.

Player A	Player B
Right Bow Step Right Ward Off	Right Bow Step Right Ward Off

Right Bow Step Left Ward Off	Right Bow Step Left Ward Off
Left Bow Step Left Ward Off	Left Bow Step Left Ward Off
Left Bow Step Right Ward Off	Left Bow Step Right Ward Off

These are the basic positions used in the initial training of Circling Hands. This is not as simple as it sounds and once players become familiar with the technique, the art then develops to other levels and no true Tai Chi Chuan player ever stops playing with this part of the form since it encompasses all the principles of the art and the very basic building block. This form will be discussed in the Tui Shou volume extensively.

San Shou is the actual application of Tai Ch'i Chuan as a fighting system. The basics are to learn the strikes and deflections and practice them repeatedly. The kicks then are developed to the Tai Ch'i Chuan model. Slow motion practice develops into full contact fighting. These are involved topics and are in the San Shou Volume. Look for all of our volumes as they become available on either our Amazon page or our web site.

The Ending

It never ends, it just takes another breath

This volume from the Internal Arts Series has focused on the Fundamentals of Tai Ch'i Chuan. There is much more to Tai Ch'i Chuan than just learning and mimicking a form. If you want to study this art there are many layers you must investigate to understand the true value of Tai Ch'i Chuan. Note that Tai Ch'i Chuan is referred to and not Tai Chi, the reason is to separate the study of the art of Tai Ch'i Chuan from the simple learning of a physical exercise. There is nothing wrong with learning Tai Chi for a daily exercise. Many people do that as can be seen in videos from the parks in China. Few venture into the depths of the art. This series is for those who wish to understand much more about the art and gain more from it in turn. Tai Ch'i Chuan covers a range of areas for investigation and hopefully you will have the patience to read each of these volumes and gain more insight and knowledge that will provide you with many gains in your life. Look for further volumes in this series on this and other parts of the Internal Arts and Health.

Volume 1 Tai Ch'i Chuan Fundamentals

Volume 2 Tai Ch'i Chuan Theory

Volume 3 Tai Ch'i Chuan - Playing the Form

Volume 4 Tai Ch'i Chuan Tui Shou

Volume 5 Tai Ch'i Chuan San Shou

About the Author

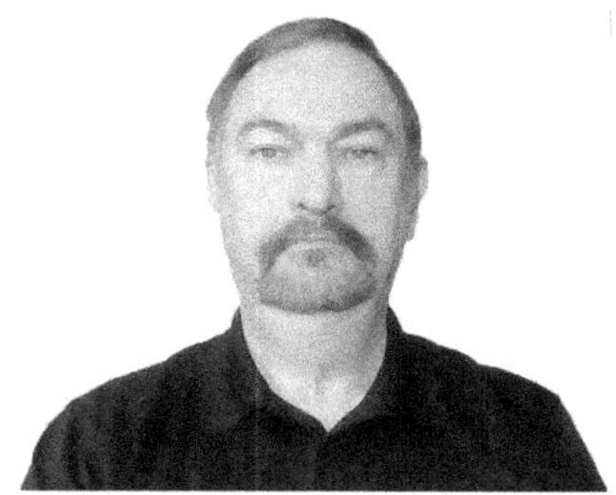

Robert George Downey (Sifu Bob) studied meditation and the martial arts most of his life. He has been a dedicated student of meditation and Internal Arts since 1970. His study started with a wide variety of systems and then focused on the Internal Arts. Sifu Bob has developed an understanding of their associated practices – meditation, Qigong, and Traditional Chinese medicine - that leads to increased skills in the arts and improved health. He has studied extensively with Grandmasters Chen and Liang. He studied and practiced Taoist Arts, Tibetan Buddhism, and Zen Meditation. He has been teaching martial arts, meditation and Qigong since the 1980's and is a co-founder of South Shore Internal Arts Association, a martial arts school that has presented seminars in the Internal Arts since the 1970's. Sifu Bob currently runs Golden Flower Internal Arts and teaches private lessons. His practice includes Tai Chi Chuan and Bagua, meditation and Qigong practice, teaching and writing every day.

Golden Flower Internal Arts

Mail

Notes

1 Player – the term play is used throughout the volumes of Golden Flower. This is in respect to the use of this term to indicate the activity by the Chinese. No one perform or does Tai Ch'i Chuan. Tai Ch'i Chuan is played. Think about the difference.

2 Break Bone Soup – Yes this is now the in soup but it has been used for centuries to heal bodies. It is simple to make. Bones are cooked in water until soft. This leaches out the nutrients from the bones. Do not add salt at this time. Ginger is frequently added since it is an herb that allows energy to flow. Remove the bones and cool. Remove excess fat. This is a base for any number of soups and herb concoctions. Look on our site for full recipes.

3 Blood and Lymph vessels transport waste – these two flows are essential for providing first nutrients and capability to combat infections with appropriate cells. While performing these functions the fluid also picks up the waste products and takes it to the filtering organs.

4 Daoyin Volume of Golden Flower provides the exercises to exercise the spine in a safe manner.

5 Tan Tien – A location below the navel and in the middle of the body that is considered a main energy center in the body.

6 Diaphragm Bending – The diaphragm actually increases the space in the thoracic cavity by tightening and pushing the abdominal organs downward. This creates space and a vacuum for the lung to fill with air.

7 Rice Cooker – A concept in the Tai Ch'i Chuan philosophy that uses the imagery of the Chinese Rice Cooker with a fire below and the stream creating the Ch'i to power the body. A more detailed description is in the Golden Flower Qigong volume.

8   Tui Shou – Also called pushing hands. This is a two p[layer practice that allows the development of the finer aspects and principles of Tai Ch'i Chuan as a martial art.

9   Drawing Silk – Those who unwind the silk cocoons learn that there is an art that requires the smooth and continuous flow of energy to keep the thread unwinding and not breaking. Tai Ch'i Chuan uses the same principle when moving through the form to keep the internal energy flowing naturally.

10 Player is used through all of the Golden Flower Internal Arts Volumes to describe the practitioner of Tai Ch'i Chuan. See number one above.

11 Engram – The mind is like a computer and contains programs for repetitive tasks. These are referred to as engrams. When you repetitively perform a movement the mind develops and refines these movements so that the player can perform the movement without consciously thinking of each part of the movement.

12 Energy Channels - The body has channels through which the energy that powers the movements flows. These channels are able to grow and get stronger with the movements of Tai Ch'i Chuan and Qigong practice. These are frequently referred to as the sinews. A full discussion of these channels is in the Tai Ch'i Chuan Theory Volume.

13 Four Fluids – the four fluids are blood, lymph, air and electrical/chemical

14 Golden Flower Internal Arts publishes a number of volumes that develop the understanding of the principles of the Internal arts.

15 Flow to the head is the spinal fluid. This is the transport of both nourishment and waste in the body. Increases this flow adds vigor to the brain and the body.

16 There can be a slight movement – the opening and closing of the joints but there is no up and down of the legs. This loses the power of

compression. Further discussion of this is in the other Tai Ch'i Chuan volumes.

17 Synovial fluid is like the oil in the car. The oil keeps the metal from wearing out the engine parts. The Synovial fluid does the same for the joints of the body. It also keeps the cartilage that covers the meeting sections of bones in the joint from deteriorating.

18 Rice Pot – See rice cooker above

19 Form Volume will provide full movements and practices for the practice of Tai Ch'i Chuan. Focus will be on the Grandmaster Chen short form with other information included.

20 Void – A void is a part of the body that is not protected by muscle or bone. They are many of differing sizes and are targets in a martial art.

21 Third nail is home – In Grandmaster Chen's system of Three Nails the third nail is the heel. It is used as a place to rest and drain energy from the body. When an action is completed frequently the heel is used as player moves to the next position.

22 Muddy Pellet – A name given by the Taoists to the back of the head. It is muddy since it is considered the hardest part of the body to get the energy flowing through it.

23 Straight line allows the spine to use its force in an efficient manner without any torque from the action injuring the body; this is like taking the kinks out of a hose to allow complete water flow.

24 Neutralization options – The body can move back and then turn to negate an attack. It can also segment the body to allow the attack to fall on nothing while still maintaining the player position. A complete explanation is in the Tui Shou Volume.

25 Channels vs meridians – Acupuncture Meridians are not the same as the energy channels used for the power that is applied in an attack.

26 Cerebral Spinal fluid – Keeping the flow of this fluid is vital for good health. The practice of Tai Ch'i Chuan and many Qigong sets uses the bodies pumping action to increase the flow of this fluid that provides nourishment and waste removal from the brain.

27 Fixed and floating ribs – The body has two types of ribs. The fixed ribs are attached to the spine and the breast bone. The floating ribs are attached to the spine and end in free space.

28 Fifth Heart – A concept from the horse industry. The Hands and Feet have a tissue that can fill with blood like a sponge. When the hands close or the feet have weight put on them the blood is pushed out through the compression and pushes the blood up the veins to the heart. This gives a heart in each hand and foot making 4 and the original makes 5.

29 Walking variations -There are many techniques to add to the walking routine. Backward walking, cross step weight transfers and other techniques. All are discussed in the San Shou volume.

30 Breath exchange process – The gas exchange process takes place in the inflating lungs. If the lungs are not totally inflated on a regular basis the remaining alveoli can fill with waste gases which are not expelled and can cause illness.

31 Internal Breathing process is very simple yet the inner workings and mental imagery requires a lot of understanding and practice. Start with just gentle in and out breathing. You will find the breaths for the form in the form volume and in the theory volume the technical details will be explored.

32 Standing Practice – A great exercise and a quality Qigong practice is the basic standing exercises. This is so essential to the development in the Internal Arts that a complete volume is dedicated to this practice.

33 Macroscopic Circulation is the greater full body circulation of energy from the ground over the head and back to the ground. This is discussed

in the Qigong volume and will be revisited in many of the other volumes. Practice just the simple thought of the energy flowing up and down and do not try to move anything until a full understanding of the whole process and the issues that may develop.

34 Movement – a stance and a posture make up a movement in the form

35 Series – Golden Flower Internal Arts has divided the series into volumes directed at specific parts of the Arts. A complete list of each volume can be found on our Amazon site.

36 Break the back – when the hand or arm moves behind the back this is called break the back. The body consists of the 4 corners – 2 shoulder and 2 hips. This creates a plane. Any activity of the arms behind that plan does not allow for the use of the whole body energy. This can be seen in this movement or when someone draws back to throw a punch. It does not follow the principles of Tai Ch'i Chuan.

37 See above

38 White Crane Spreads Both Wings – This is a movement that has been added by Grandmaster Chen to his long form. It is an original movement in Tai Ch'i Chuan but seldom practiced. It is discussed in the form volume.

39 Three Forms – this is considering the William Chen Short form, the Professor's form also short and either one of the long forms listed.

40 Again remember that the long form from either Grandmaster Liang or Grandmaster Chen can be used. They differ slightly on the naming and the movements.

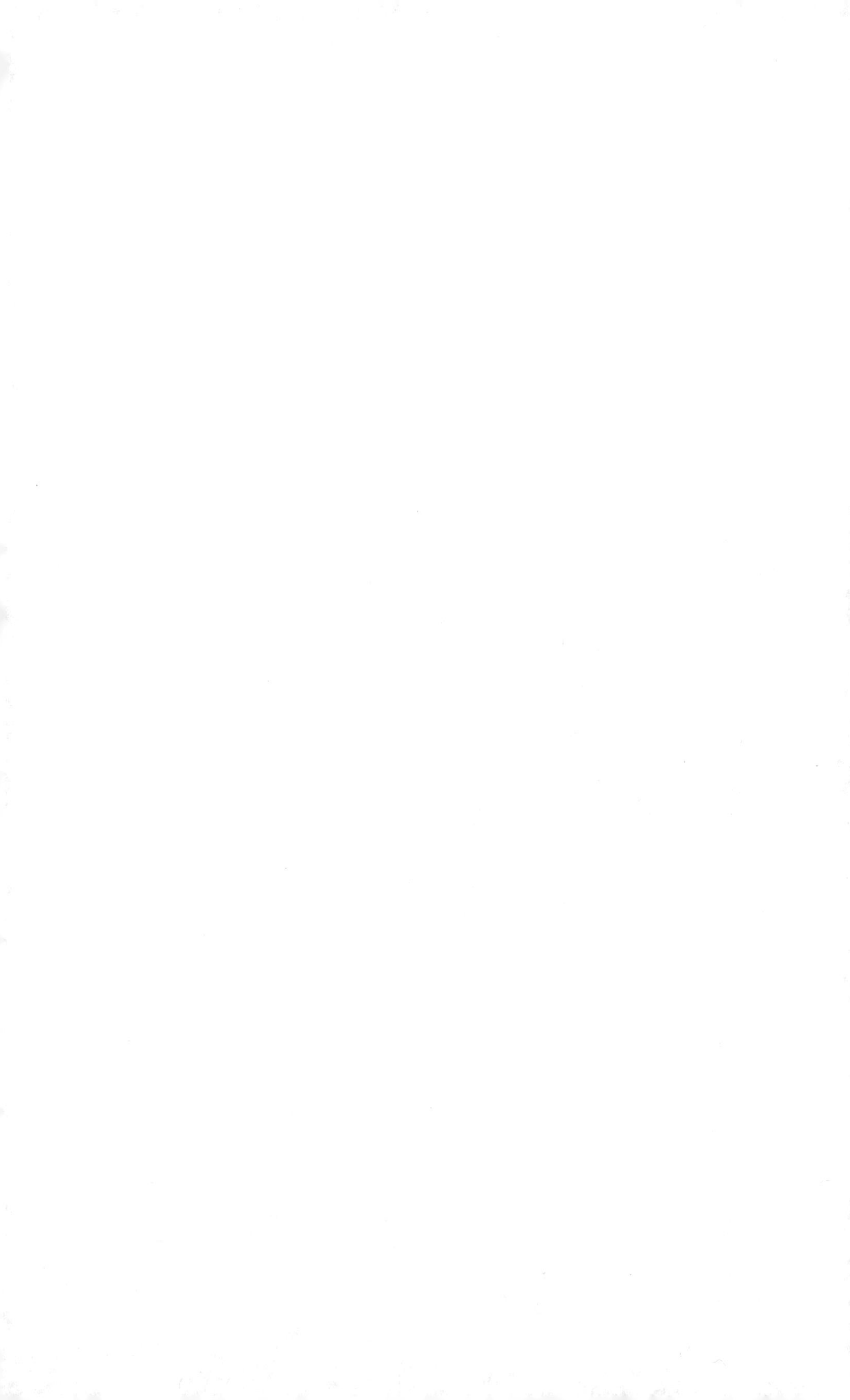